T0331223

Real-World Evidence in a Patient-Centric Digital Era

Real-world evidence is defined as evidence generated from real-world data outside randomized controlled trials. As scientific discoveries and methodologies continue to advance, real-world data and their companion technologies offer powerful new tools for evidence generation. **Real-World Evidence in a Patient-Centric Digital Era** provides perspectives, examples, and insights on the innovative application of real-world evidence to meet patient needs and improve healthcare, with a focus on the pharmaceutical industry.

This book presents an overview of key analytical issues and best practices. Special attention is paid to the development, methodologies, and other salient features of the statistical and data science techniques that are customarily used to generate real-world evidence. It provides a review of key topics and emerging trends in cutting-edge data science and health innovation.

Features:

- Provides an overview of statistical and analytic methodologies in real-world evidence to generate insights on healthcare, with a special focus on the pharmaceutical industry
- Examines timely topics of high relevance to industry such as bioethical considerations, regulatory standards, and compliance requirements
- Highlights emerging and current trends, and provides guidelines for best practices
- Illustrates methods through examples and use-case studies to demonstrate impact
- Provides guidance on software choices and digital applications for successful analytics

Real-World Evidence in a Patient-Centric Digital Era will be a vital reference for medical researchers, health technology innovators, data scientists, epidemiologists, population health analysts, health economists, outcomes researchers, policymakers, and analysts in the healthcare industry.

Chapman & Hall/CRC Biostatistics Series

Recently Published Titles

Simultaneous Global New Drug Development
Multi-Regional Clinical Trials after ICH E17
Edited by Gang Li, Bruce Binkowitz, William Wang, Hui Quan, and Josh Chen

Quantitative Methodologies and Process for Safety Monitoring and Ongoing Benefit Risk Evaluation
Edited by William Wang, Melvin Munsaka, James Buchanan, and Judy Li

Statistical Methods for Mediation, Confounding and Moderation Analysis Using R and SAS
Qingzhao Yu and Bin Li

Hybrid Frequentist/Bayesian Power and Bayesian Power in Planning Clinical Trials
Andrew P. Grieve

Advanced Statistics in Regulatory Critical Clinical Initiatives
Edited By Wei Zhang, Fangrong Yan, Feng Chen, and Shein-Chung Chow

Medical Statistics for Cancer Studies
Trevor F. Cox

Real-World Evidence in a Patient-Centric Digital Era
Edited by Kelly H. Zou, Lobna A. Salem, and Amrit Ray

For more information about this series, please visit: www.routledge.com/Chapman--Hall-CRC-Biostatistics-Series/book-series/CHBIOSTATIS

Real-World Evidence in a Patient-Centric Digital Era

Edited by
Kelly H. Zou
Lobna A. Salem
Amrit Ray

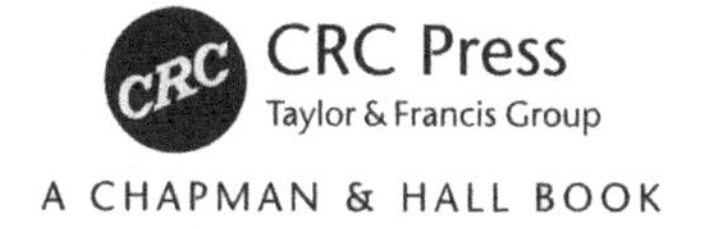

A CHAPMAN & HALL BOOK

First edition published 2023
by CRC Press
6000 Broken Sound Parkway NW, Suite 300, Boca Raton, FL 33487-2742

and by CRC Press
2 Park Square, Milton Park, Abingdon, Oxon, OX14 4RN

CRC Press is an imprint of Taylor & Francis Group, LLC

ISBN: 9780367861810 (hbk)
ISBN: 9781032303628 (pbk)
ISBN: 9781003017523 (ebk)

DOI: 10.1201/9781003017523

Publisher's note: This book has been prepared from camera-ready copy provided by the authors.

Contents

Preface

Real World Evidence and Digital Innovation to Combat Noncommunicable Diseases

Kelly H. Zou,[1] Lobna A. Salem,[1] Joseph P. Cook,[1]
Anurita Majumdar,[2] and Amrit Ray[3]
[1]Viatris, [2]GlaxoSmithKline, [3]Principled Impact, LLC

Why do Real-World Evidence and Digital Technologies Matter?

The Food & Drug Administration (FDA) defines Real-World Data (RWD) as "the data relating to patient health status and/or the delivery of healthcare routinely collected from a variety of sources" (FDA, 2022a). Healthcare facilities routinely collect medical and patient data and electronically record them when patients use their facilities. Such recording continues even after patients leave the healthcare facility. The gathering of these data provides the healthcare community with a significant amount of useful medical and patient information.

Real-world evidence (RWE) "is the clinical evidence regarding the usage and potential benefits or risks of a medical product derived from analysis of RWD" (FDA, 2022a). As the name suggests, RWE provides scientific and clinically relevant real-world information to improve medical care for patients globally (FDA, 2018).

Digital technologies support access to quality healthcare in a number of ways and for separable purposes. They include electronic healthcare ("eHealth"), which covers a range of electronic technologies applied to healthcare and relates principally to the application of computers. Mobile health ("mHealth") relates to the subset of eHealth that uses mobile technologies to share information over the radio waves. Artificial intelligence combines systems that mimic human intelligence and robust datasets to propel healthcare with new insights across early diagnosis, prevention, and treatment.

Randomized controlled trials (RCTs) often do not address the complex intersection of many diseases and comorbid conditions, which are patient centric and require us to find alternate ways of getting evidence to support such need gaps.

NonCommunicable Diseases around the World

Noncommunicable diseases (NCDs) are the leading cause of death around the world. The devastation of a "silent killer" has increasingly become a critical global health burden. Despite the overwhelming burden of NCDs, RCTs address disease entities and not NCDs holistically (KFF, 2019).

The problem of NCDs cannot be overstated, according to the World Health Organization (WHO). NCDs account for 71% (41 million) of global deaths each year, nearly 44% of which are attributable to cardiovascular disease (CVD), including stroke and ischemic heart disease; 22% to cancer; 9% to chronic respiratory disease; and 4% to diabetes (Noncommunicable Diseases, WHO). Around 30% of these deaths are premature, occurring before the age of 70 years, and it is documented that every two seconds one person between the ages of 35–75 would die prematurely from NCDs. CVD is often categorized as a disease of wealthy, industrialized societies. Yet with increased urbanization and changing lifestyles over the years, over 75% of CVD-related global deaths occur in low- and middle-income countries (LMIC), while in high-income countries (HICs), cancer is particularly prevalent. Europe, for example, with one-eighth of the world population, has one-quarter of all cancer cases. Three-hundred million people have chronic respiratory diseases worldwide, and this number is increasing. Likewise, the number of people with diabetes has increased nearly fourfold since 1980. With the coronavirus disease of 2019 (COVID) pandemic disproportionately impacting people living with NCDs, many patients suffered NCD-related comorbidities blurring the lines between what are known widely as communicable versus noncommunicable diseases. The pandemic has added to the complexity of the public health challenge and the difficulty in providing an effective solution to the growing NCDs burden. Hence, understanding NCDs with the objective of effective control should be a key consideration in the healthcare agendas of governments, multilateral organizations, and the private sector (WHO, 2022; KFF, 2019; Pan American Health Organization [PAHO], 2022).

A sobering reality of NCDs is not only their mortality burden but also their major contribution to morbidity and disability. To make things more complicated, NCDs associated with the greatest morbidity and disability burden differ from those responsible for the greatest risk of mortality. For example, mental illness and chronic pain are recognized as key drivers of NCD-related morbidity and disability with a heavy economic burden but are not considered major contributors to mortality.

The overall economic burden of NCDs continues to increase and it has been estimated that a cumulative US $47 trillion in economic output will be lost to NCDs between 2010 and 2030 (The US Government and Global Non-Communicable Disease Efforts). In the United States (US) alone, the costs of managing chronic diseases are projected to total US $4.2 trillion yearly by 2023. To understand how to combat the burden of NCDs, there needs to be a thorough understanding of the underlying causes of NCDs. Two major factors contribute to the burden of NCDs, namely disease-related and healthcare system-related factors. Disease-related factors include environmental and behavioral risk factors, some of which are modifiable, such as tobacco use and unhealthy diet, while others are non-modifiable, such as CVD that is more common in men than women.

For healthcare system-related factors, the lack of patient awareness and empowerment, along with limited access to well-trained primary care physicians to manage NCDs, leads to an overall gap in the integration/coordination of care across the patient journey. Despite the technology revolution seen in many other sectors, technology in healthcare has not been leveraged to provide adequate solutions to the challenges posed by NCDs. Gaps in leveraging big data are revealing signs of the struggles to take advantage of what technology and diverse data sources (drug registries, healthcare data) can offer. Analyses of these data sources with the patient with chronic diseases at their center has the ability to generate meaningful learnings that could contribute significantly to address the data gap in NCDs' burden.

Real-World Evidence in NonCommunicable Diseases

Given the negative impact of NCDs on patients' and their families' lives, we recommend the use of data-driven methods (e.g., RWE) for understanding global healthcare policymaking with a view to address the burden and impact of NCDs broadly. We believe that RCTs tend to focus on less diverse patient populations to compare therapies, which leaves gaps in the evidence (FDA, 2022b). Hence, we recommend the use of RWE to complement the evidence, which would help in obtaining timely data for actionable insights and enabling informed decision making for NCD policies. There are also ways to consider external control arms and synthetic control arms (FDA, 2019).

There are multiple ways that RWE can help address the NCD crisis, including in relation to prevention, epidemiology, diagnosis, risk-assessment, patient journey analysis, treatment choices, and prognosis. Using evidence generated from multiple sources in the real world and from multiple markets, we can map patient journeys to better understand adherence to therapies and to measure outcomes. In NCDs, in particular, it is common for patients to have multiple comorbid conditions and diseases that overlap. Therefore, quantitative and qualitative information can help evaluate patients' diagnoses, therapies, and prognoses holistically and comprehensively. Furthermore, a beyond NCD-only approach can also be considered with approaches that seek to address social determinants of health, integrated care models, and innovative technologies such as telemedicine to improve patient outcomes and access to medicines.

Social Determinants of Health

Global evidence suggests that social determinants of health account for a major part of the distribution of disability and mortality from NCDs (Healthy People 2030, U.S. Department of Health and Human Services). Currently, NCDs still cannot be effectively addressed without addressing the social inequalities that impact NCDs and their risk factors.

The prevention of NCDs requires intersectoral partnerships and collaborations to effectively address the conditions that give rise to NCDs, and to implement policies that support people to minimize their exposure to modifiable risks. Indeed, the WHO Commission on Social Determinants of Health calls for integrated action across all sectors.

To address the issues of social inequalities in health and its impact on the mortality and morbidity of NCDs, a coordinated approach through robust, adequately resourced, and empowered partnerships and frameworks for NCD prevention and control that strongly engage other relevant sectors is essential to improve awareness, screening, diagnosis, access to medications, and control in NCDs in the LMICs. It is vital that health systems in LMICs ensure equitable access to preventative, acute, and chronic care to support health equity and health rights.

Dynamics of Evolving Information for Value-Based Care

RWE offers a wealth of information to improve population health by identifying additional risks, costs, and benefits. RWE has long been used in the post-marketing safety monitoring of new medicines, as even though clinical trials provide important information on a drug's efficacy and safety, it is "impossible to have complete information" at the time of a new medicine's approval (FDA, 2022b; 2022c). In the same way, evidence about a medicine's reimbursement value to patients will expand and evolve over its market life and support changes to private and public reimbursement strategies using the best available evidence (Solle et al., 2020). Finally, technologies related to the gathering and analyzing of data continue to evolve as well, making available new types of evidence.

Adaptive licensing, in some forms, recognizes the lack of complete information and even embraces it. In such processes, evidence requirements and access are balanced over time to allow sensible access while further evidence is developed that might allow for the license to be supplemented to extend access (Eichler, 2012). Learning is undertaken, recognizing there is some residual uncertainty, and further phases of data generation and analysis facilitate further learning. Supplemental indications and adjustments to existing indications are intended to be iterated over time. "FDA will work with its stakeholders to understand how RWE can best be used to increase the efficiency of clinical research and answer questions that may not have been answered in the trials that led to the drug approval, for example how a drug works in populations that weren't studied prior to approval" (FDA, 2018).

What is the role of a pharmaceutical company in patient-centric care as an amplifier for the voices of caregivers and other healthcare stakeholders?

Different teams within the pharmaceutical industry harness RWE to work with internal and external partners, and to amplify the voices of multiple healthcare stakeholders. For example, for medical affairs, RWE can help enable partnerships with agencies making authorization decisions, help provide academic and physician associations with new evidence to develop treatment guidelines and recommendations, and provide enriched content for medical education. For regulatory affairs, RWE can help prioritize product registration processes, support regulatory authorities' data queries, and provide insights for label expansion. Moreover, for commercial, RWE can provide information to support pricing and reimbursement decisions by payors, support business strategies and business development plans, enable commercial and due diligence assessments, make growth plans for informed decision-making, and deliver insights for market access.

About the Book

This book on RWE and digital innovation provides an overview of concepts, methodologies, and examples to generate patient-centric insights. Specifically, it exemplifies NCDs as the leading cause of death and disability worldwide. It examines an array of topics such as bioethics, ethics, regulations, and compliance in big data. It highlights emerging and current trends and guidelines for best practices. It illustrates methods through examples and use-case studies to demonstrate impact. Finally, it provides guidance on data and digital applications for analytics.

References

Eichler HG, Oye K, Baird LG, Abadie E, Brown J, Drum CL, Ferguson J, Garner S, Honig P, Hukkelhoven M, Lim JC, Lim R, Lumpkin MM, Neil G, O'Rourke B, Pezalla E, Shoda D, Seyfert-Margolis V, Sigal EV, Sobotka J, Tan D, Unger TF, Hirsch G. Adaptive licensing: taking the next step in the evolution of drug approval. Clin Pharmacol Ther. 2012 Mar;91(3):426-37.

Food & Drug Administration. Framework for FDA's Real-World Evidence Program. 2018. www.fda.gov/media/120060/download (Accessed on March 30, 2022).

Food & Drug Administration. Breaking Down Barriers Between Clinical Trials and Clinical Care: Incorporating Real World Evidence. into Regulatory Decision Making: Speech by Scott Gottlieb, M.D. 2019. www.fda.gov/news-events/speeches-fda-officials/breaking-down-barriers-between-clinical-trials-and-clinical-care-incorporating-real-world-evidence (Accessed on March 30, 2022).

Food & Drug Administration. Real-World Evidence. 2022a. www.fda.gov/science-research/science-and-research-special-topics/real-world-evidence (Accessed on March 30, 2022).

Food & Drug Administration. Step 5: FDA Post-Market Drug Safety Monitoring. 2022b. (www.fda.gov/patients/drug-development-process/step-5-fda-post-market-drug-safety-monitoring) (Accessed on March 30, 2022).

Food & Drug Administration. FDA Offers Guidance to Enhance Diversity in Clinical Trials, Encourage Inclusivity in Medical Product Development. 2020. www.fda.gov/news-events/press-announcements/fda-offers-guidance-enhance-diversity-clinical-trials-encourage-inclusivity-medical-product (Accessed on March 30, 2022).

Department of Health and Human Services, Office of Disease Prevention and U.S. Department of Health and Human Services, Office of Disease Prevention and Health Promotion. Social Determinants of Health. 2022. https://health.gov/healthypeople/objectives-and-data/social-determinants-health (Accessed on March 30, 2022).

KFF. The U.S. Government and Global Non-Communicable Disease Efforts. 2019. www.kff.org/global-health-policy/fact-sheet/the-u-s-government-and-global-non-communicable-diseases (Accessed on March 30, 2022).

Pan American Health Organization. NCDs and COVID-19 2022. www.paho.org/en/ncds-and-covid-19 (Accessed on March 30, 2022).

Solle JC, Steinberg A, Marathe P, Gray TF, Emmert A, Abel GA. Patients as experts: characterizing the most relevant patient-reported outcomes after hematopoietic cell transplantation. Bone Marrow Transplant. 2020 Jan;55(1):242-244

World Health Organization. Noncommunicable diseases. 2022. Available at: www.who.int/news-room/fact-sheets/detail/noncommunicable-diseases (Accessed on March 30, 2022).

Contributors

Joseph P. Cook
Shaantanu Donde
Danute Ducinskiene
Ewa Filipowska
Kim Gilchrist
Tarek A. Hassan
Yvonne Huang
Joseph S. Imperato,
Jim Z. Li
Olive Jin
Gabriel Jipa
Anurita Majumdar
Diana Morgenstern
Eleanor Panico
Corinne Pillai
Amrit Ray
Mina Riad
Salman Rizvi
Jean-Pascal Roussy
Jorge Enrique Saenz
Lobna A. Salem
Urooj Siddiqui
Joan van der Horn
Zhi Xia Xie
Wei Yu
Claudia Zavala
Kelly H. Zou

About the Editors

Kelly H. Zou, Ph.D., PStat® is Head of Global Medical Analytics and Real World Evidence, Viatris. She is an elected Fellow of the American Statistical Association and an Accredited Professional Statistician. Previously, at Pfizer Inc, she was Vice President and Head of Medical Analytics & Insights; Senior Director of Real-World Evidence; Group Lead of Methods & Algorithms and Analytic Science Lead; and Senior Director of Statistics. She was Associate Professor of Radiology at Harvard Medical School, as well as Director of Biostatistics at its affiliated teaching hospitals. She was Associate Director of Rates at Barclays Capital. Dr. Zou is the Vice Chair of the Methods and Data Council of AcademyHealth and Methodologies Working Group, Digital Medicine Society. She has published extensively on both clinical and methodological topics and 160 peer-reviewed publications. She has served on the editorial board of *Significance, Statistics in Medicine, Academic Radiology*, and *Radiology*. She was the theme editor of "Mathematical and Statistical Methods for Diagnoses and Therapies" in "Philosophical Transactions of the Royal Society A." She has authored *Statistical Evaluation of Diagnostic Performance: Topics in ROC Analysis, Patient-Reported Outcomes: Measurement, Implementation and Interpretation*, and *Statistical Topics in Health Economics and Outcomes Research* published by Chapman and Hall/CRC, Taylor & Francis. She also authored a book chapter in *Leadership and Women in Statistics*.

Lobna A. Salem, MD, MBA is the Regional Chief Medical Officer for North, Europe, Japan, Australia & New Zealand at Viatris. Previously, she was Chief Medical Officer, Developed Markets, Upjohn, a Division of Pfizer Inc. Lobna has more than 25 years of experience of global experience in the biopharmaceutical industry across various leadership positions that spanned global, regional and local roles in various parts of the world including both high-, middle-, and low-income countries. In addition to her broad medical affairs experience Dr. Salem has held different cross- functional experience in clinical development, regulatory as well as commercial roles in the pharmaceutical industry. Before joining industry Lobna was a physician in the National cancer institute in Egypt. Dr Salem is a key advocate and expert in strategies to combat NCD (Non communicable disease) across the globe and has been forging strong partnerships with different stakeholders to drive solutions in this highly unmet public health need. As an expert in the medical affairs field Lobna has been working across industry to evolve the role of medical affairs in the pharma industry to be the strong voice that bridges industry and healthcare ecosystem. Lobna has been recognized for driving innovation across Research and Development in Legacy Upjohn, a Division of Pfizer Inc. Dr Salem is a Clinical Pathologist/ Hematologist by training;

she received her medical degree from Cairo University, Egypt, her MBA from Edinburgh Business School in the United Kingdom (UK), and MSc from Hibernia College in Ireland.

Amrit Ray, MD, MBA is a globally experienced industry leader, physician researcher, and biopharmaceuticals expert. Dr. Ray is Managing Partner at Principled Impact, LLC. His passion is advancing medical breakthroughs and championing healthcare access for patients. He has over 20 years of healthcare experience and has held three C-level roles of increasing responsibility at major companies, leading up to 3,500 professionals in 90 countries. Previously, Dr. Ray was Global President, Head of R&D and Medical, and Executive Leadership Team member at Pfizer Upjohn where he oversaw all aspects of research, Phases I-IV development, regulatory, safety, and medical affairs worldwide. He served as the company's most senior decision-maker and spokesperson on patient matters. Before joining Pfizer, he was the global Chief Medical Officer for pharmaceuticals at Johnson & Johnson. He earned Immunology and Medical degrees from Edinburgh Medical School, and an MBA from Dartmouth College's Tuck School of Business. Following antibody bench research at Sir Joseph Lister Labs, obesity clinical research at the Mayo Clinic, and clinical training at Edinburgh Royal Infirmary, he began his career serving as a hospital doctor delivering patient care in the UK's National Health Service. In industry, Dr. Ray has championed the development and launch of several new medicines including in Oncology, Immunology, Neuroscience, Cardio-Metabolism, and other areas. Dr. Ray has wide experience as an independent board director and private equity senior advisor. He serves as an Executive in Residence in bioethics at Columbia University, a Visiting Professor in the Faculty of Medical Sciences, Newcastle University, UK, and a board director at the EveryLife Foundation for rare diseases.

Disclaimer

Kelly H. Zou, Lobna A. Salem, and Joseph P. Cook are employees of Viatris, merged between Upjohn, a Division of Pfizer, and Mylan. Anurita Majumdar is an employee of GSK and a former employee of Upjohn, a Division of Pfizer, and Viatris. Amrit Ray is an employee of Principled Impact, LLC and a former employee of Upjohn, a Division of Pfizer, and Viatris. The views expressed are the authors' own and do not necessarily represent those of their employer or employers. The authors appreciate the editorial support from Arghya Bhattacharya and Aswin Kumar A of Viatris.

1

Real-World Evidence Generation

Joseph S. Imperato, Joseph P. Cook, Diana Morgenstern, Kim Gilchrist, Tarek A. Hassan, Jorge Saenz, and Danute Ducinskiene
Viatris

CONTENTS

1.1 Types of Real-World Data and the Generation of Real-World Evidence

Healthcare facilities routinely collect medical and patient data and electronically record them when patients use their facilities. Measurements of blood pressure, prescribed medications, and patients' medical symptoms and diagnosis are a few examples. This electronic data recording continues even after patients leave the healthcare facility, especially when they need to get a prescription filled in a pharmacy or have medical claims processed by an

DOI: 10.1201/9781003017523-1

insurance company or government agency. The electronic gathering of these data not only helps healthcare facilities to improve the quality of and efficiency in delivering medical care, but also provides the healthcare community with a significant amount of useful medical and patient data. Patients themselves can also provide helpful electronic data via other channels, such as using social media, joining patient registries, or via wearable devices. Cumulatively, these records, known as Real World Data, can be used to find ways to improve the quality and effectiveness of medical treatments provided to patients everywhere, now and into the future. The Food & Drug Administration (FDA) defines real-world data (RWD) as "data relating to patient health status and/or the delivery of health care routinely collected from a variety of sources," and "RWD can come from a number of sources." In fact, the electronic recording of medical and patient data is happening all over the world (FDA, 2022).

Healthcare providers (doctors, hospitals, etc.), universities, government agencies, and biopharmaceutical and healthcare companies conduct research using RWD to investigate new ways to improve the quality of patient healthcare. They then share research findings with healthcare providers (HCPs) around the world. The findings from the analysis of RWD is called "real-world evidence" (RWE), which the FDA defines as "clinical evidence regarding the usage and potential benefits or risks of a medical product or intervention derived from analysis of RWD," and "RWE can be generated by different study designs or analyses, including but not limited to, randomized trials, including large simple trials, pragmatic trials, and observational studies (prospective and/or retrospective)." (FDA, 2022).

The FDA's definition of RWD provides that effectively RWD are all electronic patient information not collected in a clinical trial. According to FDA (2022), RWD can be but not limited to the following types:

- Electronic health records (EHRs)
- Claims and billing activities
- Product and disease registries
- Patient-generated data including in home-use settings
- Data gathered from other sources that can inform on health status, such as mobile devices

EHRs, generally a collection of electronic medical records (EMRs), refer to patient information electronically gathered at doctors' offices, clinics, and hospitals, etc. As healthcare practices began to use standard technology to document patient information, service providers were able to electronically record and collate data, providing the foundation for syndicated EMR and EHR data services like the The Health Improvement Network (THIN), which is a large European database of fully anonymised and non-extrapolated

Electronic Health Records collected at the physicians' level (Cegedim, 2022). The electronically recorded information included diagnoses, medicines, tests, treatment plans, and physicians' notes, delivering a longitudinal view of patient health over time.

Similarly, medical and prescription claims were submitted electronically and processed by government and commercial payers, giving rise to commercially available claims data services from companies such as Optum, Premier Healthcare Database, and IQVIA. These databases also provide financial insights into the medical treatments that can be leveraged for population health and health economic and outcomes research (HEOR). Health surveys gather and deliver insights from patients, providers, or individuals in the general population on health status, healthcare utilization, treatment patterns, and healthcare expenditures. Finally, patients themselves provide information via patient registry databases, wearable devices or participating in social media dialogues (Katkade et al. , 2018).

Having provided an overview of the type of information that exists on over a billion patients spanning at least ten years, let us now focus on methods being used to turn data into RWE. Advancements in technology and data processing methodologies have significantly improved our ability to perform efficient analysis on the massive amount of complex RWD ("big data"), creating powerful information used for health promotion, prevention, and improving healthcare quality for patients globally. In addition, RWD sources have information recorded over many years, enabling us to analyze several years of repeated patient healthcare observations including prescriptions, symptoms, test results, etc., known as longitudinal studies. The ability to perform statistical and data analysis continues to evolve and improve rapidly as computer storage and processing power advances. Later, we discuss the data analytic methodologies and processing techniques prevalent in the industry today, for example, the advancements in statistical based data analysis, machine learning (ML), artificial intelligence (AI), and natural language processing (NLP) that is driving much of the innovation in the RWE-generation area.

Here, we examine how the creation of RWE has delivered advancements in healthcare across domains, such as improving the ability for medical professionals to diagnose patients and enhance patient treatment guidelines. The dramatic increase in the availability of RWD globally has significantly expanded our ability to understand the impact of diseases on patients and the burden of diseases on society. Health organizations around the world such as the Centers for Disease Control and Prevention (CDC) and World Health Organization (WHO) partner with local governments, other public institutions, hospitals, and other treatment facilities to electronically record and disseminate this information so that they can be collated and reported. As a result of this work, these organizations can now provide insights into key epidemiological information such as disease prevalence i.e., the percent of the population with the medical condition), incidence (i.e., the frequency of new cases occurring yearly), and patient demographics in a country, region, or population (Hedberg and Maher, 2018). In fact, Clarivate sources RWD from many areas including public and patient databases and literature searches to deliver the Incidence & Prevalence Database (IPD) database providing incidence and prevalence information for most diseases across population demographics for most countries around the world (Incidence & Prevalence Database, 2022). This is only one of the many arenas that a healthcare professional can obtain valuable insights on patient health and the burden of diseases globally.

One of the initial phases of providing healthcare to a patient is the diagnostic phase where a patient's health, symptoms, tests, etc., are reviewed by a health care professional (HCP) with the goal of providing a diagnosis. The diagnostic process requires the HCP to assess all the known patient information and, based on their experience, knowledge, and existing guidelines, make a diagnosis. RWD has been evaluated to review longitudinal patient information to better develop and expand guidelines for diagnosing diseases. This type of retrospective data can be used to look at the symptoms and tests of patients prior to diagnoses to improve understanding of the disease, a process that can be very beneficial for diagnosing diseases that can be very challenging and complex. Fibromyalgia, a disorder characterized by widespread musculoskeletal pain, is an example of this type of disease in that the symptoms – widespread pain, fatigue, sleep and mood issues, and cognitive difficulties – are generalized and overlap with other diseases (Mayo Clinic, 2022). A recent study of 2,529 fibromyalgia patients with 79,570 observations or clinical visits was evaluated. The study applied a combination of artificial intelligence (AI) and machine learning (ML) algorithms to administrative claims data from the ProCare Systems' network of Michigan Pain Clinics to identify four groupings of fibromyalgia patients based on patient pain characteristics and other symptoms. These groupings have proved to be very helpful with developing diagnostics and treatment guidelines (Davis et al, 2018).

Having made the diagnosis, the HCP will once again leverage his or her years of experience and medical guidelines to make treatment recommendations. Treatment guidelines are critical components of the healthcare process. Traditionally, the initial guidelines are defined as a result of the randomized controlled trial (RCT) performed to assess the efficacy of a treatment for a disease. The advances in RWE have provided effective ways for guidelines to be continually reviewed and enhanced globally based on EHRs obtained in real-world settings. One example of this is a retrospective non-interventional study in Taiwan that was published in 2019 and that leveraged the claims database of Taiwan's National Health Insurance. The goal was to evaluate the impact of patient treatment adherence to prescribed statins in patients with established atherosclerotic cardiovascular disease (ASCVD) for secondary prevention of subsequent cardiovascular events. The study evaluated 185,252 patients with post discharge statin prescriptions, and there were 50,015 ASCVD re-hospitalizations including 2,858 in-hospital deaths during the seven years of the study. The study demonstrated that patients with good medicine adherence and persistence were at a statistically significant lower risk of re-hospitalization or in-hospital deaths than patients with a less persistent or compliant state (Chen et al. 2019). This study provided RWE on not only the efficacy of the established treatment guidelines but also the importance of patient adherence. Treatment adherence is an important topic that we will discuss in much greater detail later in the chapter.

We continue to give insights into all the valuable ways that RWE is being leveraged across the healthcare community. However, several known challenges and limitations exit when harnessing RWE. The first concern is incomplete or inaccurate data, as well as the overall data quality of RWD sources since most of the time the data is not initially captured with the intention of utilizing the information for research or future analysis. This concern continues to lessen, though, as the technology and applications improve, and the overall quantity of RWD enables analysts to remove poor data and still have enough information to perform studies. The second area of concern, and the most substantial, is that these types of retroactive and non-interventional studies are viewed as being limited in their ability to provide a causal inference like the gold standard: RCTs (Katkade, Sanders and Zou, 2018). Much more detail will be provided on this topic later in the book. Even with this limitation RWE continues to provide incredibly valuable insights. During the coronavirus disease 2019 (Covid-19) crises in 2020, electronic data sources were instrumental in helping to understand and document the epidemiology and patient demographics of the disease. Review of these data sources helped identify comorbid conditions and other factors that would increase the risk of a more severe response to the disease. Some of the comorbid conditions that increased health outcome risks were hypertension, diabetes, and obesity, etc. These insights provide extremely valuable information to the healthcare community in identifying patients at greater risk and with treatment guidelines (Hasan et al. 2020). In subsequent chapters, we discuss the additional way that RWE is being leveraged and the many opportunities for RWE's expanded, future use.

1.2 The Evidence Hierarchy and Importance of RWE/Digital

Evidence should be built from reliable data that reflects the type of information needed to answer the questions in which one is interested. Reliable data can be assessed over a number of attributes. Agmon and Ahituv (1987) offer three reliability concepts: internal, relative, and absolute. If data are reliable, they should reflect what an ordinary person would expect and be suited to the proposed purpose. At a fundamental level, the data should represent some "truth." It would not be helpful to have the data present some version of reality that bore no resemblance to it.

There are rules of thumb captured in hierarchies of evidence based on the source data that have wide appeal. Conventionally, the RCT is considered a "gold standard," with its artificial structure designed to limit the role of untested factors in affecting the outcomes. However, sometimes the question is less precise than what measurable effect a proposed treatment can have on selected patients in a controlled environment and asks what sorts of outcome await the population at large when this treatment reaches the market. Of course, this later question may be difficult, if not impossible, to answer without observing what happens when the treatment actually reaches the market. Moreover, those outcomes may change as market conditions change over time.

The difference in the sort of question one asks drives what sort of evidence is appropriate. Questions that regulators typically ask with respect to a new molecule's authorization are designed to help ensure that the product actually does something and that the risks of any negative side effects are offset by the expected benefits. When the Kefauver-Harris Drug Amendments to the Federal FD&C Act were passed in 1962, the requirement for evidence that had to consist of controlled studies was "a revolutionary requirement" (Meadows 2006). This helped mark the beginning of an evidentiary evolution for medicines, that would later go on to include cost-effectiveness analyses for reimbursement that would add consideration of a trade-off between insurer-based costs and monetized clinical benefits. Over time, a greater role for the patient's perspective and patient-reported outcome measures would be added as well as social determinants effecting population health. Considerations used in reimbursement decisions continue to expand and include substantial variance in the elements of value considered in the approach depending upon the assessor or reimburser (Lakdawalla et al., 2018).

As data have become more plentiful and ubiquitous, their use is more common. People develop more comfort with its use and greater confidence in evidentiary results derived from it. Techniques advance to analyze data of different types and to greater effect, as discussed elsewhere in this volume. The importance in healthcare relates, at least in part, to the complex nature of the marketplace for healthcare. We are all patients, at least prospectively, even if one is of that rare type who is never sick a day in their life. However, we often need expert advice from physicians, and in some instances, special authorization (e.g., prescription medicine) or services (e.g., surgery), in pursuit of treatments to improve our health. Beyond that, most people either arrange or have arranged for them some measure of risk sharing through insurance, which can also act has a collective purchasing agent, whether through public or private insurers. Of course, pharmacists and nurses and others play their roles as well and look to RWD and RWE.

Within these complex relationships, there is a raft of uses for RWD and RWE. The healthcare community is using these data to support coverage decisions and to develop guidelines and decision support tools for use in clinical practice (FDA, 2022). "Reviews of the literature and publicly available HTAs and reimbursement decisions suggested that HTA bodies and payers have varying experience with and confidence in patient reported outcome (PRO) data. Payers participating in the survey indicated that PRO data may be especially influential in oncology compared with other therapeutic areas (Brogan et al., 2017). The pharmaceutical and medical devices industries use evidence developed from real world sources to support clinical trial designs and observational studies to support the discovery and licensing process for new treatments (FDA, 2022). Of course, regulatory use plays a key role. The FDA monitors post-marketing safety and adverse events using real world data and evidence (FDA, 2022). With the advent of the 21st Century Cures Act, the FDA embraced the use of real world evidence for at least the expansion of approved uses for products that already have some area for which they have marketing authorization (FDA, 2022). The use of RWE in regulatory decisions is not limited to pharmaceuticals, and there are also several examples of RWE used in medical device decisions (FDA, 2021).

While evidence of some type is interesting to many different stakeholders, the evidence is not always being sought to help inform the same question. Regulators are interested in evidence that helps in weighing the tradeoff between clinical benefit and risk for the patient. That regulators hold RCTs up as a "gold standard" for evaluating these linked questions of clinical efficacy and safety is widely recognized (Franklin and Schneeweiss 2017). In contrast, insurers and HTA agencies ask a different question although one that still considers these clinical factors. These stakeholders look to discern whether they are financially better off given the costs of introducing a treatment and using a monetized measure of the clinical changes to patients. While both involve some measurement of the benefits relating to one or more clinical changes in patients, each of these questions are different. However, concerns have been expressed about the validity of RWE, suggesting that some stakeholders would like as much as possible to be derived from clinical trials (FDA, 2021).

RWE involves a variety of tasks. With so many alternative datasets available and such a wide array of stakeholder perspectives, judging the feasibility of alternative datasets and selecting the most appropriate alternative available can be an undertaking of its own. Of course, the protocol must be developed with the precise nature of the data being used in mind as well as the measures that one wishes to obtain and their planned use and audience. Such might take the form of advice in the clinical trial program to best prepare for later work, as well as considerations over the lifecycle of a product or treatment to include post-hoc trial analyses and meta analyses.

Market observers will note the recent push for a shift from "volume" to "value" in healthcare paired with expressions of interest in new contracts that reimburse healthcare providers and suppliers based on the quality of the outcomes they foster, rather than the utilization of their goods and services. RWE can be used to adjudicate contracts where the level of reimbursement or the price is a function of some selected outcome. A clinical outcome can be derived from claims data or EHRs or captured purposefully in some form of patient registry or digital application. In principle, this could help more closely approximate an efficient market, assuming that the outcome closely correlates with patient preferences.

Perhaps one of the earliest hierarchies for evidence comes from 1979 and the Canadian Task Force on the Periodic Health Examination, although it would be revisited by others over time and often presented as a pyramid (Mulimani 2017). The spirit of having RCTs at or near the top of the pile and working down to expert opinions based more broadly and more on experience.

> I: Evidence obtained from at least one properly randomized controlled trial.
>
> II-1: Evidence obtained from well-designed cohort or case-control analytic studies, preferably from more than one centre or research group.
>
> II-2: Evidence obtained from comparisons between times or places with or without the intervention. Dramatic results in uncontrolled experiments (such as the results of the introduction of penicillin in the 1940s) could also be regarded as this type of evidence.
>
> III: Opinions of respected authorities, based on clinical experience, descriptive studies or reports of expert committees.
>
> The periodic health examination. Canadian Task Force on the Periodic Health Examination 1979

From 1979 to today, this idea of ranking evidence or placing evidence in a hierarchy would continue to evolve and be refined with further considerations. For example, in Ho et al. (2008), the authors discuss evidence hierarchy in a pyramid form and note that in applying evidence one must consider the circumstances and, however well-suited RCTs are to evaluations of the efficacy of new treatments in a controlled experimental setting, such designs are not always feasible or appropriate for other important questions. More recently, a new interpretation of the pyramid by Murad et al. (2016) explored the interpretation of systematic reviews and meta-analyses of RCTs in the pyramid. Rather than seeing them as the top of the pyramid, leap-frogging over RCT by leveraging the power or multiple RCTs, they offered the notion that these kinds of studies were really a lens of interpretation of the rest of the pyramid, with RCTs still at the highest tier. Moreover, they suggest that, given that other factors beyond the design of the study producing the evidence can affect its certainty, the lines between tiers (designs) are blurred or "wavy" rather than sharply denoting a change in rank as one moves from one layer to another.

1.3 Real-World Evidence and Its Relationship to Population Health, Epidemiology, and Observational Studies in Population Health

Population health was just becoming its own concept in 2003 when Kindig and Stoddard defined it as the health outcomes of a group of individuals, including the distribution of such outcomes within the group as evaluated by health outcomes, patterns of health determinants, and policies and interventions that link these two. (Kindig and Stoddard, 2003) Since then and through the dawning of "big data" many have worked to understand and shape the idea of population health, including tackling its distinction from public health. According to the CDC, public health works to protect and improve the health of communities through policy recommendations, health education and outreach and research for disease detection and injury prevention. Public health can be defined as what "we as a society do collectively to assure the conditions in which people can be healthy." On the other hand, population health provides "an opportunity for health care systems, agencies and organizations to work together in order to improve the health outcomes of the communities they serve" (What Is Population Health? Online Public Health).

This potential for public-private partnership is key to answering real world health questions, especially if improving health broadly is viewed as an interdisciplinary, customizable approach that allows health departments to connect practice to policy for change to happen locally. Using this approach, non-traditional partnerships among different sectors of the community – public health, industry, academia, health care, local government entities, etc. – can be leveraged to help achieve positive health outcomes, with focus as needed on allocation of health resources across the population (What is Population Health? Population Health Training in Place Program (CDC, 2022).

RWE is particularly germane to population health partnerships. Access to real world data may be the reason different sectors come together in the first place, or the resulting evidence may form the foundation for future health-improving initiatives. RWE to support healthcare decision making and to further population health is derived from a multitude of data sources and methods of analysis. Observational and epidemiologic studies are among the key tools used to flesh out the role and value of interventional and preventative strategies utilizing medicines, vaccines and/or devices; an understanding of these tools, along with an appreciation for the concepts of public and population health is essential when considering what is "real."

As a starting point, the science of epidemiology systematically studies the distribution and determinants of health-related states and events. Epidemiology studies are generally conducted in human populations to understand whether there is an association or causal relationship between observed or adverse health effects and exposure to a substance (What Are Epidemiology Studies? ToxTutor. The National Institutes of Health's (NIH) National Library of Medicine (NLM).) Different study designs provide different ways of gathering the information sought (Aschengrau and Seage 2008). Landmark epidemiologic investigations include the relationship of smoking to lung cancer, and the identification of risk factors associated with cardiovascular disease as identified with the Framingham population study in Massachusetts.

In contrast, observational study is a type of study in which individuals are observed or certain outcomes are measured (National Cancer Instittue, 2022). No attempt is made to affect the outcome (for example, no treatment is given.) As such, observational data are the essence of "real world." Observational studies are non-experimental in nature, and thus their role and validity has been a controversial topic in the literature (Collins and Bowman 2020). Nonetheless, observation-based studies can suggest important areas for RCTs, hypothesis generation or clarify our understanding of patient experience. They can do so by utilizing various designs including case report or case series, ecologic, cross-sectional (i.e., a prevalence study), case-control and cohort studies (Kumar and Khan 2014).

Formal observational and epidemiologic studies, however, are not the only sources of RWE. The International Statistical Classification of Diseases and Related Health Problems (ICD) system (WHO, 2022) provides another important aspect of the transactional recording of healthcare. ICD purpose and uses are as follows:

- Allows the systematic recording, analysis, interpretation and comparison of mortality and morbidity data collected in different countries or regions and at different times
- Ensures semantic interoperability and reusability of recorded data for the different use cases beyond mere health statistics, including decision support, resource allocation, reimbursement, guidelines and more

An evaluation and management process is core to every patient encounter and is supplemented by Current Procedural Terminology (CPT). These elements are recorded together as an "encounter" incorporating time spent with the patient, the specific health condition, and associated comorbidities (e.g., International Classification of Diseases 10th Revision [ICD-10]). These features describe the services provided to a particular individual within the healthcare system. The recording of each healthcare encounter and the associated data elements are utilized to complete the healthcare transaction between providers, insurers, and patients. These data, in aggregate, form the elements utilized as the language between healthcare entities and the "real world" transactional experience of patients engaging in the healthcare process.

For an evaluation of patient populations, it would be difficult to develop a research cohort designed prospectively utilizing the target population, condition, and intervention to understand the resultant health outcomes. Observational research has bridged this dilemma with new research datasets which link transactional information, disease classification, co-morbidities, interventions, and therapeutics to understand health outcomes. Electronic data capture of the patient journey has expedited and further clarified the patient journey in a longitudinal framework by linking data sets with individual patient records across healthcare entities (laboratory, pharmacy, specialist, diagnostic, etc.).

Because an individual patient journey is not always feasible to construct, an alternative has been the focus on populations of individuals based on condition, diagnosis, and overall health. It has allowed for larger cohorts with similar conditions to be evaluated with respect to provider engagement, co-morbidities, diagnostic, and treatment modalities. Examples of populations evaluated for overall health patterns and co-morbidities are the cardiovascular conditions and the potential outcomes of coronary atherosclerosis in those with diabetes mellitus. These sorts of evaluations foster a learning healthcare environment; for example, as these conditions were studied, it was noted that those with diabetes had more significant overall vascular disease, leading to the key learning that diabetes mellitus alone is a risk factor for cardiovascular disease (CVD).

As previously mentioned, the value and role of data generated via observational and/or epidemiological study has been debated. RCTs evaluate specific populations with rigorous controls through inclusion and exclusion criteria – an "ideal" population, to inform understanding of efficacy or adverse experiences. However, more complete understanding of a population's health, requires additional evaluation of the variability in healthcare delivery, outcomes, and participation (Gerard and Cohn 2021, Hernan 2021). Epidemiological evaluation of variables for age (e.g., the elderly), gender and cultural differences and co-morbidities unique to individuals and sub-populations can help to tell the story. Such evaluation may also allow for observations of human behavior – the willingness to adhere to interventions, treatments, and the measurement of response. While it may not always be able to define actionable outcomes, epidemiologic evaluations can inform future hypotheses and strategies to address the "real-world" observations and the population health at a local, regional, or global level. Electronic health records and research in an automated manner can help fill in informational gaps and expedite our ability to identify patterns and trends in care delivery and outcomes in order to further our understanding about the population overall.

Population health is truly established in partnership between the public and healthcare practice communities, data scientists and academic partners who together evaluate epidemiology, make real world observations and record public health disease and its outcomes. This combination of scientific and data analytic approaches to large and subset groups can come closest to simulating the real-world experience and describing the current health state of the population. Harnessing the 'ying and yang' of observational studies and big data sources, such as electronic health records, is the current evolution which will inform population health. Knowing where the population health is in the moment will better inform the next hypotheses and clinical studies to bring improvements in health outcomes.

1.4 Randomized Controlled Trials and Pragmatic Clinical Trial Optimization Using RWE

For medical affairs, the regulatory approval and launch of a new novel intervention is always a great opportunity to lead a conversation with the healthcare professionals and payers about this new intervention.

Medical affairs are the front runners to share the knowledge about the efficacy and safe use of the new intervention from the outcomes of the explanatory phase III RCTs that estimate the efficacy as well as the safe use which led to the approval of the new intervention.

After approval, medical affairs are also participating in guiding the design and supervision of the phase IV observational studies, which reflect the real-life experience of the efficacy and tolerability of the new intervention.

This new opportunity comes with challenges, as healthcare professionals and payers usually have some legitimate questions, which might not be sufficiently answered based on the nature of the explanatory studies which are usually designed under optimized conditions with an ideal situation in highly selected group of patients within certain age, gender, ethnicity, other organs function and with certain level of adherence and health literacy usually in specialized clinical research centers (Ford and Norrie, 2016).

Exclusion of other patient profiles or criteria make it a little bit difficult to answer questions and queries about the external validity and generalizability of the effect of the new intervention in other patients' groups not tested in phase III RCTs.

For more than 70 years, RCTs have been universally established as the gold standard for informing the clinical community about the efficacy and safety of new intervention in a highly selected group of patients with specific medical condition/disease (Knottnerus et al., 2017; Christian et al., 2020).

An RCT is a way of doing impact evaluation in which the population receiving the programme or policy intervention is chosen at random from the eligible population, and a control group is also chosen at random from the same eligible population. It tests the extent to which specific, planned impacts are being achieved (White et al., 2014).

It has been widely acknowledged that for most of the new interventions, the immediate evidence after the regulatory approval is insufficient to fully inform physicians and policy-makers on the efficacy and safe use of the new intervention in a wider group of patients in the real life clinical practice and there is a need to generate a real world evidence on the practical use of the new intervention in a more sophisticated patients' profile (Zuidgeest et al., 2017).

In 1967 Schwartz and Lellouch, described for the first time the new concept about the pragmatic clinial trials (PCTs), which can guide clinical practice, healthcare professionals and policy decision by providing evidence for the adoption of the new intervention into real-world clinical practice and also described their differences from the explanatory trials, which experiment a physiological or clinical hypothesis (Schwartz and Lellouch, 1967).

Improving the quality of care especially with a relatively new intervention, including approaches to improve its effectiveness through a real-world practice is critical.

A pragmatic randomized controlled trial (pRCT) includes a population that is relevant for the intervention, a control group treated with an acceptable standard of care, and outcomes that are meaningful for patients. It must be conducted and analyzed at a high standard of quality (Ford and Norrie, 2016).

The need for the pragmatic randomized controlled trials (pRCTs) design that reflect the reality of clinical practice, enhance external validity and give confidence in the clinical applicability and generalizability of the clinical trials results (Knottnerus et al., 2017).

To ensure that the trial design decision matches the intended outcomes of the trial the PRECIS & PRECIS-2 (PRagmatic Ex-planatory Continuum Indicator Summary) tools were developed (Thorpe et al., 2009; Loudon et al., 2015).

Firstly, the PRECIS tool was developed to identify and quantify trial characteristics that can differentiate between pragmatic and explanatory trials to assist academic and industry researchers in designing pragmatic clinical trials (Thorpe et al., 2009). The PRECIS was a tool with 10 domains to design clinical trials on a continuum of explanatory attitude (ideal situation) to more pragmatic attitude (usual care)

1. Participant eligibility criteria
2. Flexibility of experimental intervention
3. Experimental intervention — practitioner expertise
4. Flexibility of the comparison intervention

5. Comparison intervention — practitioner expertise
6. Follow-up intensity
7. Primary trial outcome
8. Participant compliance with "prescribed" intervention
9. Practitioner adherence to study protocol
10. Analysis of the primary outcome

Secondly, in 2015, the PRECIS-2 tool (Figure 1.1) was published with only nine domains including three new ones (recruitment, setting, and organization), each scored on a 5-point Likert continuum (from 1=very explanatory "ideal conditions" to 5=very pragmatic "usual care conditions") (Loudon et al., 2015).

The multidimensional structures in PRECIS and PRECIS-2 tools will help in defining the type of clinical trials (either explanatory or pragmatic) based on the design of the trial to maximize the usefulness to potential users (Thorpe et al., 2009 & Loudon et al., 2015).

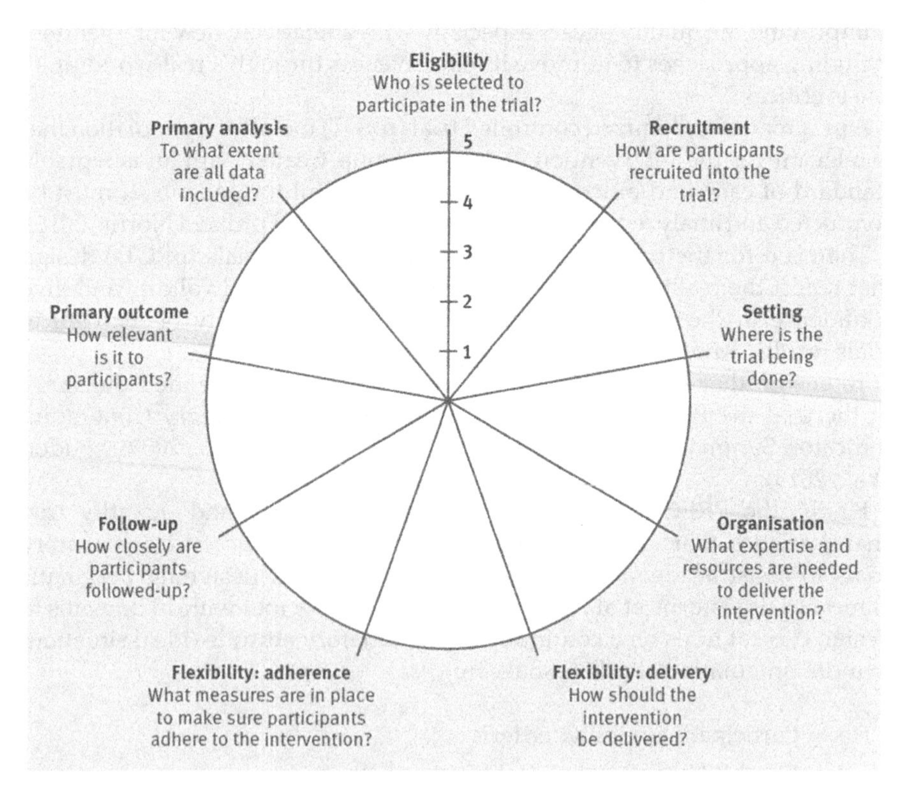

FIGURE 1.1
The Pragmatic-Explanatory Continuum Indicator of Summary @ (PRECIS-2) wheel.

The pRCTs should not replace the explanatory randomized controlled trials as each trials' design should address legitimate needs in the clinical trials continuum.

Both pragmatic and explanatory clinical trials have their strengths and weaknesses and they can be complementary to each other. Pragmatic trials can be beneficial in hard to reach population as well as in rare diseases with a very limited number of patients. RWD obtained from the EHRs and disease and drug registries could be helpful when the explanatory randomized controlled trials might not be feasible (Ramsey L, 2020).

Some considerations for designing and conducting the pragmatic randomized controlled trials:

1.4.1 Ethics

1. The standard written informed consent for clinical research should not be altered unless there is a clear necessity. The updated informed consent or waivers should be approved by the relevant ethics committee before use.
2. Risks and benefits of participation in pragmatic RCTs should be discussed with participants despite they might not be different from the usual care.
3. There is a need for regulatory oversight if the pragmatic RCTs will be used for approving a new intervention or changing policies.
4. Equity of access to pragmatic RCTs and responsibilities should be defined during the design of the trial.
5. The definition of usual care may be different across geographies as well as by time and should be standardized to avoid questioning the external validity (Nicholls et al., 2019).

1.4.2 Randomization

Randomization in explanatory RCTs is critical to ensure that the baseline characteristics are similar. The balance between treatment groups is critical in a randomized controlled trial to ensure that the observed outcome is interpreted as the causal effect of the treatment.

As in explanatory RCTs, randomization in the pRCTs can also be ensured at the patient level or at the cluster level e.g., at the research sites, clinic or at the investigator level (Gamerman et al. 2019).

The pRCT is an RCT, which accommodate clinical reality with key pragmatic design elements:

1. Real clinical practice population
2. Classical clinics and hospitals rather than specialized research centers

3. Real clinical practice active comparator instead of the placebo arm
4. Measure relevant clinical outcomes to patients, health care providers as well as policymakers. Obtaining data from electronic heath records as well as real-time data from self-care devices can simplify the data reporting (Gamerman et al. 2019).

Another kind of new suggested randomization design is the cohort multiple randomized controlled trials (cmRCTs), developed to solve some challenges for the pRCTs.

Researchers can use a large observational cohort of patients who are recruited and used as a multiple trials facility: each randomized controlled trial uses random selection of some participants (not random allocation of all); and "patient centered" information and consent are applied (Relton et al. 2010).

1.4.3 Blinding

Blinding in RCTs is always desired for testing the new interventions to ensure that there is no bias from the subjective factors in the evaluation of the desired outcomes. Sometimes blinding is not feasible for ethical reasons when we compare a new intervention (drug) versus surgery.

One of the factors that increases the internal validity of the study results, beside the randomization, is the blinding as part of the clinical trial design. Blinding in pRCTs is usually not feasible as a comparison of the new intervention versus the standard care will break this kind of blinding. Possible strategies to compensate for the unblinding is to focus on hard end points, use adjudicated committee and statisticians who are blinded during the trial conduct (Gamerman et al. 2019).

There is a great need to generate high-quality, larger, more generalizable, and more cost-effective pragmatic randomized controlled trials (pRCTs) using real-world data.

Digital data capture, including electronic consent; and linkages between data sources can foster support clinical research and promote high-quality clinical care (Curtis et al., 2019).

1.5 Improving Adherence via Data-Driven Methods

Adherence to medication is one of the most complex behaviors of patients. Non-adherence to a therapeutic regimen can result in negative outcomes and may be aggravated in populations with chronic diseases due to the prolonged duration of multiple drug treatments.

Lack of adherence to medication is a growing concern as it is increasingly associated with negative health outcomes and a higher cost of care. Addressing the burden of non-adherence requires a collaborative, patient-centered approach that considers individual patient needs and results in smart interventions that combine high technology with high contact. Lack of adherence increases the cost burden for all major stakeholders in the health system, as the resulting deterioration in health may require the use of more costly services, such as those found in the acute care or emergency care system. This creates a vicious cycle of deteriorating health outcomes and rising healthcare costs.

Despite many years of research and studies, non-adherence to medication is still very common. According to the WHO (2003), 50% of patients deviate from their chronic treatments. Nonadherence to medication leads to poor health outcomes, increased use of health services, and increased direct and indirect costs, jeopardizing the efficacy of evidence-based therapies (Cutler et. al, 2018). In a recent meta-analysis, lack of adherence to medication was found to be associated with hospitalization for all causes (adjusted odds ratio 1.17, 95% CI 1.12–1.21) and mortality (the good adherence was associated with a 21% reduction in the risk of long-term mortality compared with non-adherence to medication; adjusted hazard ratio 0.79, 95% CI 0.63–0.98) in older people (Walsh et al, 2019). Therefore, non-adherence is an important determinant of individual health. At the population level, it also seriously affects public health and the economy.

Unfortunately, this problem is growing. A major reason for this is the impressive demographic change we are facing in the twenty-first century. Although the impact is global, it is particularly shocking in Europe.

Median age of the EU-27 population expected to increase by 5.1 years between 2019 and 2100, and the number of people aged 80 years and over projected to rise to 60.8 million in EU-27 by 2100. European Union (EU)-27 population (Eurostat, 2022). Longer life expectancy results in an increase in the prevalence of chronic non-communicable diseases and multimorbidity (i.e., the coexistence of two or more chronic diseases in an individual). This leads to the frequent use of complex therapeutic regimens and creates fertile ground for non-compliance (Wong et al., 2014).

To prevent non- or low adherence, we need to know its main drivers. The WHO developed a model and grouped the factors that affect adherence into five main sets: health system-related factors, therapy-related factors, condition-related factors, patient-related factors, and socioeconomic factors (WHO, 2003). Based on this model, multiple interventions targeting non-adherence have been designed and tested, but only a few have been successful.

Taking medication is a complex behavior and various determinants affect it at the individual level. Consequently, a uniform intervention is unlikely to solve the problem in all cases. On the other hand, there is growing evidence supporting the use of innovative digital solutions as an effective way to manage non-adherence (Car et al., 2017). Successful examples include web-based education and monitoring programs (Linn et al., 2011), clinical decision support systems using EHR data to produce alerts (Bailey et al., 2019), mobile technologies, applications that provide various combinations of patient follow-up, adherence education and facilitation (Hamine et al., 2015). Thanks to digitization, non-adherence can also be accurately measurable on a large scale due to the availability of large healthcare databases. However, we still lack widely accepted basic standards for measuring and managing adherence based on big data. Well, it is necessary to change this scenario through the development of skills and the creation of capacities to analyze big data (Priority Recommendations of the Heads of Medicines Agencies (HMA) and European Medicines Agency's (EMA) joint Big EMA, 2022). We require robust standards for big data format and analysis to assess, uniformly present, and compare medication adherence patterns across studies and thus aid scientific research and clinical practice.

Digitization is a great opportunity. To date, digital solutions have been widely used outside of healthcare, but have only recently begun to be used in the medical field where they offer great promise towards more efficient care. To accelerate this process, in 2018, the European Commission developed a plan for the digital transformation of healthcare. The plan is based on three pillars: (1) ensure data access and exchange; (2) connect and share health data for research, faster diagnosis, and better individualized healthcare services and health outcomes; and (3) strengthen citizen empowerment and individual care through digital services (European Commission, 2022).

The digitization of the healthcare sector creates an opportunity to use big data analytics tools and methods to assess non-adherence, improve clinical practice, and promote the use of personalized interventions. Routinely collected prescribing and dispensing information, which is available from HCE, pharmacy dispensing databases, health insurance claims systems, and national health system registries, allows a more comprehensive exploration of the relationship between adherence and health outcomes. Thus, big data can represent a powerful and relatively low-cost resource for investigating important public health problems in real-life settings, including the prevalence of non-adherence, its drivers, and the consequences of non-adherence. Big data can also be used to provide information to design new interventions and focus on both prevention and management of non-adherence. In addition, big data enables research on an unmatched scale, covering large populations. However, uniform and accepted standards of adherence measurement for big data are still lacking. The Big Data Collection does not have a uniform format or structure for measuring adherence. Therefore, to build a solid evidence base for the management of adherence in clinical settings, it is necessary to standardize the estimation of adherence and facilitate the appropriate use of these standards (Dima, Allemann and Dediu 2019).

Without standard metrics, the same data can lead to diverse results, as clearly described in the study by Malo et al. (2017), which found different mean values of adherence and proportions of patient's adherent when using the proportion of medication possession versus the proportion days covered. To date, there have been numerous studies on adherence, using various approaches to data analysis, leading to mixed results. The International Society for Research in Pharmacoeconomics and Results (ISPOR) has made some attempts to introduce standards for assessing adherence in big data. The ISPOR Medication Adherence and Persistence Special Interest Group developed recommendations for the assessment of initial medication adherence (Hutchins et al., 2015) and proposed a checklist for medication adherence studies using retrospective databases (Peterson et al., 2007). At the same time, a systematic review of publications on adherence in older Americans identified up to 20 adherence measures with different names derived from the pharmaceutical claim data (Sattler, Lee and Perri 2013). Even more interesting, some adherence measures derived from big data are already in use to aid healthcare providers to consider long-term health outcomes. Another important question to be addressed in future standardized measures of adherence in big data is what is the subject of adherence assessment: a drug, a disease, or a patient? In other words, how to measure adherence to multiple prescription drugs for the same and/or multiple conditions in patients with multimorbidity (Kim et al., 2018). Indicators designed and widely used to assess adherence to a single drug are not necessarily valid for assessing adherence to polypharmacy regimens (Arnet et al., 2018). A recent systematic review found serious inconsistencies in the measures used to estimate adherence and persistence to multiple cardiometabolic medications (Alfian et al., 2019), while another review concluded that "there does not appear to be a standardized method for measuring adherence to multiple medications" (Pednekar et al., 2019). Certainly, more research is needed in this regard and it is particularly important given the aging of the population. In summary, the main disadvantage of the current lack of widely accepted standards for the assessment of adherence is the difficulty in comparing and interpreting the results of scientific studies. There is an urgent need to develop a uniform measurement of adherence to support research and allow real-life implementation of the study findings (Dima and Dediu 2017). This is also necessary for inter-study comparisons and fair benchmarking of interventions targeting adherence.

Big data and the development of a standardized measure of adherence can facilitate more reliable and valid research on the association between non-adherence and health outcomes. To date, there is no agreed standard on what constitutes adequate adherence. In practice, 80% is often used as the cut-off point for classifying "good adherence", but the scientific evidence for this threshold is unclear. Indeed, a systematic review investigated medication adherence thresholds in relation to clinical outcomes and found the included studies to be highly heterogeneous and was unable to confirm or reject the validity of the historical 80% cutoff threshold for adherence (Baumgartner et al., 2018). Also, many treatments are preventive, and it can take a long time to determine the therapeutic benefit of such treatments. Several interventions have been designed to prevent and manage nonadherence in real-life settings. Unfortunately, these interventions are generally underused. The lack of standardized and comparable compliance measures is one of the main barriers to the objective selection of the most effective and cost-effective interventions (Cutler et al., 2018) and the scaling-up of best practices. Only with reliable and valid measures can non- or low compliance be traced, allowing for the assessment of the long-term effects of particular interventions and the comparative evaluation of their effectiveness. Standard measures and guidelines for assessing adherence could also facilitate the introduction and assessment of the effectiveness of incentives to promote adherence at the patient, provider, and payer levels and the ability to address individual risk factors (Khan and Socha-Dietrich 2018). Standardized compliance measures employed in large data sets can also provide information on the reasons why patients are not adhering to prescription drug regimens. A review of systematic reviews identified 771 individual factor items as possible determinants of non-adherence (Kardas, Lewek and Matyjaszczyk 2013). Large data sets are useful for assessing adherence in different profiles of drug users, analyzing adherence-related factors, exploring causes of discontinuation, and comparing results in different populations. With this information, drug users most at risk of non-compliance can be identified and tailored interventions can be designed and implemented. It is extremely important to consider that the majority of current interventions address adherence use or are based on information technology (IT) solutions. However, they are not currently based on standardized measures of adherence (Khan and Socha-Dietrich 2018). Another potential technological approach to adherence prediction and evaluation is AI. With AI, big data can be analyzed both retrospectively and in real time, enabling more personalized healthcare. However, a major obstacle to AI adoption is, once again, the lack of robust operational adherence measures to adequately train algorithms.

Public health will benefit from the introduction of standardized compliance measures. Such measures will allow comparison of adherence rates within and between different countries, populations, and disease groups, allowing for comparative evaluation of interventions, better planning, and practical implementation. Increasingly, adherence to medication is accepted as a measure of the quality of medical care, as well as the quality and effectiveness of the entire health system (Khan and Socha-Dietrich 2018). On the other hand, the lack of standardized measures means that the problem of non-adherence is often overlooked in national agendas. Currently, only a few countries systematically monitor adherence. Therefore, the recent report by the Organization for Economic Cooperation and Development (OECD) calls for standardization to allow international benchmarking (Khan and Socha-Dietrich 2018).

The recent outbreak of the COVID-19 pandemic has demonstrated the extraordinary role that info epidemiology (i.e., information epidemiology) can play in treating major public health problems (Mavragani 2020). This lesson should lead us to a wider adoption of digitization as well as the faster use of big data for adherence management.

Disclaimer

Joseph P. Cook, Kim Gilchrist, Tarek A. Hassan, Jorge Saenz, and Danute Ducinskiene are employees of Viatris, merged between Upjohn, a Division of Pfizer, and Mylan. Joseph Imperato and Diana Morgenstern are former employees of Upjohn, a Division of Pfizer, and Viatris. The views expressed are the authors' own and do not necessarily represent those of their employer or employers. The authors appreciate the editorial support from Arghya Bhattacharya and Aswin Kumar A of Viatris.

References

Alfian SD, Pradipta IS, Hak E, Denig P. A systematic review finds inconsistency in the measures used to estimate adherence and persistence to multiple cardiometabolic medications. J Clin Epidemiol 2019 Apr; 108:44–53.

Arnet I, Greenland M, Knuiman MW, Rankin JM, Hung J, Nedkoff L, et al. Operationalization and validation of a novel method to calculate adherence to polypharmacy with refill data from the Australian pharmaceutical benefits scheme (PBS) database. Clin Epidemiol 2018; 10:1181–1194.

Aschengrau A, Seage GR. Epidemiology Studies. Essentials of Epidemiology in Public Health. Jones & Bartlett Publishers; 2008.

Bailey SC, Wallia A, Wright S, Wismer GA, Infanzon AC, Curtis LM, et al. Electronic Health Record-Based Strategy to Promote Medication Adherence Among Patients With Diabetes: Longitudinal Observational Study. J Med Internet Res 2019 Oct 21; 21(10)

Baumgartner PC, Haynes RB, Hersberger KE, Arnet I. A Systematic Review of Medication Adherence Thresholds Dependent of Clinical Outcomes. Front Pharmacol 2018; 9:1290.

Brogan AP, DeMuro C, Barrett AM, D'Alessio D, Bal V, Hogue SL. Payer Perspectives on Patient-Reported Outcomes in Health Care Decision Making: Oncology Examples. J Manag Care Spec Pharm. 2017 Feb; 23(2):125–134.

Car J, Tan WS, Huang Z, Sloot P, Franklin BD. eHealth in the future of medications management: personalisation, monitoring and adherence. BMC Med 2017 Apr 05;15(1).

Cegedim. THIN: The Health Improvement Network. 2022. www.cegedim-health-data.com/cegedim-health-data/thin-the-health-improvement-network (Accessed March 30, 2022).

Chen ST, Huang ST, Shau WY, Lai CL, Li JZ, Fung S, Vicki CT and Lai MS, 2019. Long-term statin adherence in patients after hospital discharge for new onset of atherosclerotic cardiovascular disease: a population-based study of real world prescriptions in Taiwan. BMC Cardiovascular Disorders, 19(1), pp.1–13.

Christian JB, Brouwer ES, Girman CJ, Bennett D, Davis KJ, Dreyer NA. Masking in pragmatic trials: who, what, and when to blind. Therapeutic Innovation & Regulatory Science. 2020 Mar;54(2):431–6.

Centers for Disease Control and Prevention. Population Health Training: PH-TIPP Overview. 2022. www.cdc.gov/pophealthtraining/ph-tipp/overview.html (Accessed on March 30, 2022).

Clarivate. Integrated patient journey: Leveraging real world data and analytics to understand patients' unmet needs. 2022. https://clarivate.com/lp/integrated-patient-journey-leveraging-real-world-data-analytics-understand-patients-unmet-needs (Accessed on March 30, 2022)

Coding for Evaluation & Management Services, Available at: www.aafp.org/family-physician/practice-and-career/getting-paid/coding/evaluation-management.html (Accessed on March 30, 2022).

Collins R, Bowman L The Magic of Randomization versus the Myth of Real-World Evidence New England Journal of Medicine 382; February 13, 2020, 7

Curtis JR, Foster PJ, Saag KG. Tools and Methods for Real-World Evidence Generation: Pragmatic Trials, Electronic Consent, and Data Linkages. Rheumatic Disease Clinics. 2019 May 1;45(2):275–89.

Cutler RL, Fernandez-Llimos F, Frommer M, Benrimoj C, Garcia-Cardenas V. Economic impact of medication non-adherence by disease groups: a systematic review. BMJ Open 2018 Jan 21;8(1)

Davis F, Gostine M, Roberts B, Risko R, Cappelleri JC and Sadosky A, 2018. Characterizing classes of fibromyalgia within the continuum of central sensitization syndrome. Journal of Pain Research, 11, p.2551.

Dima A, Allemann S, Dediu D. AdhereR: An Open Science Approach to Estimating Adherence to Medications Using Electronic Healthcare Databases. Stud Health Technol Inform 2019 Aug 21;264:1451–1452.

Dima AL, Dediu D. Computation of adherence to medication and visualization of medication histories in R with AdhereR: Towards transparent and reproducible use of electronic healthcare data. PLoS One 2017;12(4):e0174426

European Commission. eHealth. 2022. https://digital-strategy.ec.europa.eu/en/policies/ehealth (Accessed on March 30, 2022).

European Medicines Agency. Priority Recommendations of the HMA-EMA joint Big Data Task Force. 2022. www.ema.europa.eu/en/documents/other/priority-recommendations-hma-ema-joint-big-data-task-force_en.pdf (Accessed on March 30, 2022).

Eurostat. Population projections in the EU. 2022. https://ec.europa.eu/eurostat/statistics-explained/index.php?oldid=497115#Population_projections (Accessed on March 30, 2022).

Mayo Clinic, Fibromyalgia. 2022. www.mayoclinic.org/diseases-conditions/fibromyalgia/symptoms-causes/syc-20354780#:~:text=Fibromyalgia%20is%20a%20disorder%20characterized,your%20brain%20processes%20pain%20signals (Accessed on March 30, 2022).

Ford I, Norrie J. Pragmatic trials. New England Journal of Medicine. 2016 Aug 4; 375(5):454–63.

Food & Drug Administration. Leveraging Real World Evidence in Regulatory Submissions of Medical Devices. 2021. www.fda.gov/news-events/fda-voices/leveraging-real-world-evidence-regulatory-submissions-medical-devices (Accessed on March 30, 2022).

Food & Drug Administration. Real-World Evidence. 2022. www.fda.gov/science-research/science-and-research-special-topics/real-world-evidence) (Accessed on March 30, 2022).

Franklin JM, Schneeweiss S. When and How Can Real World Data Analyses Substitute for Randomized Controlled Trials? Clin Pharmacol Ther. 2017 Dec; 102(6):924–33.

Gamerman V, Cai T, Elsäßer A. Pragmatic randomized clinical trials: best practices and statistical guidance. Health Services and Outcomes Research Methodology. 2019 Mar; 19(1):23–35.

Gerard J, Cohn J. A Primer on Observational Measurement Assessment. 2016 August; 23(4): 404–413.

Hamine S, Gerth-Guyette E, Faulx D, Green BB, Ginsburg AS. Impact of mHealth chronic disease management on treatment adherence and patient outcomes: a systematic review. J Med Internet Res 2015 Feb 24;17(2).

Pérez-Jover V, Sala-González M, Guilabert M, Mira JJ. Mobile Apps for Increasing Treatment Adherence: SystematicReview. J Med Internet Res 2019 Jun 18; 21(6).

Hassan TA, Saenz JE, Li JZ, Ducinskiene D, Imperato J, and Zou KH, A Confluence of Acute and Chronic Diseases: Risk Factors Among Covid-19 Patients, 2020. www.significancemagazine.com/science/671-a-confluence-of-acute-and-chronic-diseases-risk-factors-among-covid-19-patients, (Accessed on March 30, 2022).

Hedberg K and Maher J, 2018. Collecting data. The CDC Field Epidemiology Manual, Centres for Disease Control and Prevention. www. cdc. gov/eis/field-epi-manual/chapters/collecting-data.html.com.eu1.proxy.openathens.net/journals/jamaoncology/fullarticle/2733797 (Accessed on March 30, 2022).

Hernán MA. Methods of Public Health Research - Strengthening Causal Inference from Observational Data. N Engl J Med. 2021 Oct 7;385(15):1345–1348.

Ho PM, Peterson PN, Masoudi FA. Evaluating the evidence: is there a rigid hierarchy? Circulation. 2008 Oct 14;118(16):1675–84.

Hutchins DS, Zeber JE, Roberts CS, Williams AF, Manias E, Peterson AM, IPSOR Medication Adherence Persistence Special Interest Group. Initial Medication Adherence-Review and Recommendations for Good Practices in Outcomes Research: An ISPOR Medication Adherence and Persistence Special Interest Group Report. Value Health 2015 Jul;18(5):690–699.

Clarivate. Incidence & Prevalence Database (IPD). 2022.www.tdrdata.com/(S(nt1uns5uzjlgz1rqiq3ld3yn))/Databases (Accessed on March 30, 2022).

IQVIA. Harness the power of real world data.2022. www.iqvia.com/solutions/real-world-evidence/real-world-data-and-insights (Accessed March 30, 2022).

Kardas P, Lewek P, Matyjaszczyk M. Determinants of patient adherence: a review of systematic reviews. Front Pharmacol 2013;4:91.

Katkade VB, Sanders KN, Zou KH. Real world data: an opportunity to supplement existing evidence for the use of long-established medicines in health care decision making. J Multidiscip Healthc. 2018 Jul 2;11:295–304.

Khan R, Socha-Dietrich K. Investing in medication adherence improves health outcomes and health system efficiency: Adherence to medicines for diabetes, hypertension, and hyperlipidaemia. In: OECD Health Working Papers No. 105. Paris: OECD Publishing; 2018:1–40.

Kim S, Bennett K, Wallace E, Fahey T, Cahir C. Measuring medication adherence in older community-dwelling patients with multimorbidity. Eur J Clin Pharmacol 2018 Mar;74(3):357–64.

Kindig D, Stoddart G. What is population health? Am J Public Health. 2003 Mar;93(3):380–3.

Knottnerus JA, Tugwell P. Research methods must find ways of accommodating clinical reality, not ignoring it: the need for pragmatic trials. J Clin Epidemiol. 2017 Aug;88:1–3.

Kumar R., Khan AM Types of observational studies in medical research. Research Methodology 2014: 1 (2) 154–9.

Lakdawalla DN, Doshi JA, Garrison LP Jr, Phelps CE, Basu A, Danzon PM. Defining Elements of Value in Health Care-A Health Economics Approach: An ISPOR Special Task Force Report [3]. Value Health. 2018 Feb;21(2):131–139.

Linn AJ, Vervloet M, van Dijk L, Smit EG, Van Weert JC. Effects of eHealth interventions on medication adherence: a systematic review of the literature. J Med Internet Res. 2011 Dec 5;13(4):e103.

Loudon K, Treweek S, Sullivan F, Donnan P, Thorpe KE, Zwarenstein M. The PRECIS-2 tool: designing trials that are fit for purpose. BMJ. 2015 May 8;350:h2147.

Malo S, Aguilar-Palacio I, Feja C, Lallana MJ, Rabanaque MJ, Armesto J, et al. Different approaches to the assessment of adherence and persistence with cardiovascular-disease preventive medications. Curr Med Res Opin 2017 Jul;33(7):1329–36.

Mavragani A. Tracking COVID-19 in Europe: Infodemiology Approach. JMIR Public Health Surveill 2020 Apr 20;6(2):e18941.

Meadows M. Promoting Safe & Effective Drugs for 100 Years, FDA Consumer—The Centennial Edition (January–February 2006). 2006. www.fda.gov/about-fda/histories-product-regulation/promoting-safe-effective-drugs-100-years (Accessed on March 30, 2022).

Mulimani PS. Evidence-based practice and the evidence pyramid: A 21st century orthodontic odyssey. Am J Orthod Dentofacial Orthop. 2017 Jul;152(1):1–8.

Murad MH, Asi N, Alsawas M, Alahdab F. New evidence pyramid. Evid Based Med. 2016 Aug;21(4):125–7.

Nachman A and Niv A (1987) Assessing Data Reliability in an Information System, Journal of Management Information Systems, 4:2, 34–44.

National Cancer Institute. Observational Study. 2022. www.cancer.gov/publications/dictionaries/cancer-terms/def/observational-study (Accessed on March 30, 2022).

Nicholls SG, Carroll K, Zwarenstein M, Brehaut JC, Weijer C, Hey SP, Goldstein CE, Graham ID, Grimshaw JM, McKenzie JE, Fergusson DA. The ethical challenges raised in the design and conduct of pragmatic trials: an interview study with key stakeholders. Trials. 2019 Dec;20(1):1–6.

Observational Study. NCI Dictionary. 2022. www.cancer.gov/publications/dictionaries/cancer-terms/def/observational-study (Accessed on March 30, 2022).

Pednekar PP, Ágh T, Malmenäs M, Raval AD, Bennett BM, Borah BJ, et al. Methods for Measuring Multiple Medication Adherence: A Systematic Review-Report of the ISPOR Medication Adherence and Persistence Special Interest Group. Value Health 2019 Feb;22(2):139–156.

Peterson AM, Nau DP, Cramer JA, Benner J, Gwadry-Sridhar F, Nichol M. A checklist for medication compliance and persistence studies using retrospective databases. Value Health 2007;10(1):3–12.

Premier Applied Sciences®, the Research Division of Premier Inc. Premier Healthcar Database: data that informs and performs. 2020. https://products.premierinc.com/downloads/PremierHealthcareDatabaseWhitepaper.pdf (Accessed March 30, 2022).

Priority Recommendations of the HMA-EMA joint Big Data Task Force. European Medicines Agency. 2022. www.ema.europa.eu/en/documents/other/priority-recommendations-hma-ema-joint-big-data-task-force_en (Accessed on March 30, 2022).

Ramsey SD, Adamson BJ, Wang X, Bargo D, Baxi SS, Ghosh S, Meropol NJ. Using electronic health record data to identify comparator populations for comparative effectiveness research. J Med Econ. 2020 Dec;23(12):1618–1622.

Relton C, Torgerson D, O'Cathain A, Nicholl J. Rethinking pragmatic randomised controlled trials: introducing the "cohort multiple randomised controlled trial" design. BMJ. 2010 Mar 19;340:c1066

Román-Villarán E, Pérez-Leon FP, Escobar-Rodriguez GA, Parra-Calderón CL. EIP on AHA Ontology for adherence: Knowledge representation advanced tools. Transl Med UniSa 2019;19:49–53.

Sattler EL, Lee JS, Perri M. Medication (re)fill adherence measures derived from pharmacy claims data in older Americans: a review of the literature. Drugs Aging 2013 Jun;30(6):383–399.

Schwartz D, Lellouch J. Explanatory and pragmatic attitudes in therapeutical trials. Journal of Chronic Diseases. 1967 Aug 1;20(8):637–48.

The periodic health examination. Canadian Task Force on the Periodic Health Examination. Can Med Assoc J (1979).

Thorpe KE, Zwarenstein M, Oxman AD, Treweek S, Furberg CD, Altman DG, Tunis S, Bergel E, Harvey I, Magid DJ, Chalkidou K. A pragmatic–explanatory continuum indicator summary (PRECIS): a tool to help trial designers. Journal of Clinical Epidemiology. 2009 May 1;62(5):464–75.

Traditional vs. Pragmatic: Changing the Trial Model with Real-World Evidence | 2020-01-24 | CenterWatch. Accessed August 5, 2021.

UnitdHealth Group. Optum. 2022. www.unitedhealthgroup.com/who-we-are/businesses/optum.html (Accessed March 30, 2022).

Walsh CA, Cahir C, Tecklenborg S, Byrne C, Culbertson MA, Bennett KE. The association between medication non-adherence and adverse health outcomes in ageing populations: A systematic review and meta-analysis. Br J Clin Pharmacol. 2019 Nov;85(11):2464–2478.

What Are Epidemiology Studies? ToxTutor. NIH National Library of Medicine. 2022. https://toxtutor.n lm.nih.gov/05-003.html. (Accessed on March 30, 2022).

What Is Population Health? | Online Public Health (gwu.edu). Accessed July 16, 2021.

White H, Sabarwal S and T de Hoop (2014). Randomized Controlled Trials (RCTs), Methodological Briefs: Impact Evaluation 7, UNICEF Office of Research, Florence.

Wong MC, Liu J, Zhou S, Li S, Su X, Wang HH, et al. The association between multimorbidity and poor adherence with cardiovascular medications. Int J Cardiol 2014 Dec 15;177(2).
World Health Organization. Adherence to long-term therapy: evidence for action. 2003. www.who.int/chp/knowledge/publications/adherence_full_report.pdf (Accessed on March 30, 2022).
World Health Organization. International Statistical Classification of Diseases and Related Health Problems (ICD). 2022. www.who.int/standards/classifications/classification-of-diseases (Accessed on March 30, 2022).
Zuidgeest MG, Goetz I, Groenwold RH, Irving E, van Thiel GJ, Grobbee DE, Package GW. Series: Pragmatic trials and real world evidence: Paper 1. Introduction. Journal of Clinical Epidemiology. 2017 Aug 1;88:7–13.

2

Applications of RWE for Regulatory Uses

Eleanor E. Panico, Corinne S. Pillai, Ewa Filipowska, and Kelly H. Zou
Viatris

CONTENTS

2.1 Inroduction - RWE in the Pharmaceutical Industry

Leveraging real-world evidence (RWE) has been of significant interest to pharmaceutical companies in recent years and in the US largely since enactment of the 21st Century Cures Act, which mandated the US Food and Drug Administration (FDA) to develop guidance for utilization of RWE to support regulatory processes. Opportunities exist for industry sponsors to leverage real-world data (RWD) for a variety of reasons, including adding or modifying an existing indication, adding a new population (e.g. expanding use), adding comparative effectiveness or safety information to a product label and, most commonly, further characterization of a product's safety profile.

In Deloitte's (Morgan et al., 2020) benchmarking survey, the top three areas for application of RWE across organizations today and in the next two or three years are as follows: (1) Supporting regulatory submissions and/or label expansion; (2) Informing the design of value-based contracts; (3) Comparative effectiveness research.

DOI: 10.1201/9781003017523-2

The use of RWE is even more appealing to biopharmaceutical sponsors for the following reasons:

1. Regulators are implementing initiatives of their own to drive the application of RWE in regulatory decision-making
2. There exists greater accessibility to data (clinical, biological, or structured/unstructured data sources) today than ever before
3. Significant technological advancements (e.g., AI-enabled data science) provide for more advanced data analysis

The use of RWE in observational RWD studies can involve both prospective and retrospective data collection. The FDA has listed several types of RWD as follows (Food & Drug Administration. Real-World Evidence. 2020c):

- Electronic health records (EHRs)
- Claims and billing activities
- Product and disease registries
- Patient-generated data including in home-use settings
- Data gathered from other sources that can inform on health status, such as mobile devices

In the US, the 21st Century Cures Act was designed to "help accelerate medical product development and bring new innovations and advances to patients who need them faster and more efficiently" (21st Century Cures Act, US FDA 2020). The Cures Act provides a foundation and framework within which FDA can work to modernize clinical trials and consider new approaches (e.g., use of RWD, RWE) to answering questions about medicines (pre and post-market). This act emphasizes the possibility for RWD, RWE to be used in a more standard fashion in the context of regulatory decision-making (Food & Drug Administration. Real-World Evidence. 2020c).

In a 2018 statement on FDA's new strategic framework to advance use of RWE to support development of drugs and biologics, the former FDA Commissioner, Scott Gottlieb, M.D., stated that "RWE provides us with a potential source of information that can complement, augment and expand our understanding of how best to use medical products -- improving what we know about our medical care" (06 December 2018) (Statement from FDA Commissioner). The current FDA Commisionar, Robert M. Califf, M.D., said during his confirmation hearing "to establish a system, built on electronic medical records, that can be used to more quickly confirm the benefits and risks of accelerated approval drugs" (Sutter, 2021). FDA also developed the 2019 guidance, "Submitting Documents Using Real-World Data and Real-World Evidence to FDA for Drugs and Biologics," to facilitate uniformity among regulatory submissions that include RWD and RWE as a component.

Likewise, major health authorities around the world, including the European Medicines Agency (EMA), Health Canada and the Japanese Pharmaceuticals and Medical Devices Agency (PMDA) are actively exploring ways to intergrate RWD and RWE into regulatory reviews and decisions. Both Health Canada and the PMDA have recently provided updated regulations and guidance to industry that encourage the use of RWD and the alignment among industry and regulators, providing guidance on how to use the data in submissions to avoid unnecessary review questions or delays (Baumfeld et al., 2020). In Europe, the EMA is establishing a Data Analysis and Real-world Interrogation Network (DARWIN EU), a coordination center which will deliver "real-world evidence on diseased, populations and the uses and performance of medicines" from across Europe which will be used by the EMA and national competent authorities as needed during a specific therapy's lifecycle (DARWIN EU).

2.1.1 RWE and Regulatory Success

Regulatory success is a term used often in the pharmaceutical industry to represent approval of a drug registration or acceptance of specific proposal to a heath authority to achieve some kind of objective. There exists several measures of regulatory success, and each measure is based on a probability (Weidman and Belsky 2020):

1. Probability of Technical Success (PTS) applies to the probability a given clinical trial/study will be successful based on pre-defined endpoints, feasibility, and other factors.
2. Probability of Regulatory Success (PRS) considers whether a regulatory authority such as the FDA will grant approval for a product. PRS is based on factors within the scope of regulatory affairs, which often includes evaluation of a specific health authority's perspective regarding the clinical relevance for a particular endpoint as it applies to suitability for defining efficacy in the context of an approval application for registration.
3. The overall probability of success considers both the PRS and the PTS and is calculated as $PTRS = PRS \times PTS$.

In practice, these probabilities may be estimated using company-specific, therapeutic specific benchmarks and assumptions (see, e.g., Zhou and Johnson, 2019). Imporantly, increased utilization of RWE for regulatory submissions and decision-making will facilitate the need for drug developers to adapt their understanding of regulatory risk as well as potential for regulatory success. This can be done by examining successful regulatory initiaives/approvals that utilized RWE, scrutinizing health authority guidances and collaborating closely with health authorities regarding refining best practices for using RWE in regulatory applications.

2.2 Pharmacovigilance and Safety Surveillance

Currently, the most common application of RWE in the pharmaceutical industry include routine pharmacovigilance (PV) activities and safety-monitoring of drugs (Good Pharmacovigilance Practices and Pharmaco-epidemiologic Assessment, US FDA 2015). To understand how RWE can be applied to such an activity, one must understand what routine pharmacovigilance entails in the context of pharmaceutical regulation.

Health authorities and regulatory bodies impose requirements on sponsors to monitor a drug's efficacy and safety over the course of its existence in markets globally. The characterization of a medicine year after year allows for important understanding of whether the medicine's benefit is greater than the risks of taking it. As defined by the WHO (World Health Organization. 2002), PV is defined as "the science and activities relating to the detection, assessment, understanding and prevention of adverse effects or any other drug-related problems" (What is Pharmacovigilance? WHO). It typically consists of the following components:

1. Establishing the initial/baseline safety of a drug/biologic product via clinical trial evaluation prior to registration on the market. Clinical trials typically consist of carefully selected patients on a medicine for a limited length of time in a controlled setting
2. Monitoring and surveilling safety over time via adverse event reporting and reports from the literature, which allows for looking at medicine in the context of 'real-world use,' where a larger number of patients, from all populations, may be using the medicine for longer periods of times and with other medications/environmental influences
3. Analysis of safety signals that arise over time
4. Communication of relevant safety information via updates to labeling or other means, as applicable
5. Recommending necessary regulatory actions, including labeling updates or market cessation in more serious cases

PV activities serve several purposes, including identification of rare adverse events (AEs), serious AEs (SAEs), AEs prevalent in certain populations, differences in safety for acute vs. chronic use, drug-food interactions and drug-drug interactions, misuse or abuse of a drug, and medication errors.

In the US, for example, post-marketing AE-reporting is governed by the regulation in 21 CFR 314.80 (Post marketing reporting of adverse drug experiences, eCFR) which defines an adverse drug experience as; "any undesirable event that is associated with the use of a drug in humans, whether or not considered drug-related and occurs in the course of the use of a drug product in professional practice. This may include drug overdose, drug abuse, drug withdrawal, any failure of expected pharmacologic action." This regulation requires sponsors to submit post-marketing safety reports, known as 15-day alerts for serious and unexpected adverse experience (foreign and domestic), as well as periodic adverse experience reports containing domestic spontaneous AEs that are serious/expected, non-serious/unexpected, non-serious/expected. Such reports are typically required quarterly for the first three years following a new drug launch market, and annually thereafter. These safety updates can eventually be a component of a drug application's annual NDA/IND annual report (CFR – Code of Federal Regulations Title 21). The FDA's Adverse Event Reporting System, also known as FAERS, is a fully automated computerized database designed to support FDA's post-marketing safety surveillance program for drugs and biologics (Questions and Answers on FDA's Adverse Event Reporting System (FAERS)).

In the European Union (EU), similar regulations are in place to monitor a drug's safety over time and the EMA Pharmacovigilance Risk Assessment Committee (PRAC) is responsible for assessing and monitoring the safety of human medicines. The PRAC is made up of safety experts and regulatory authorities in the EU Member States as well as healthcare professionals nominated by the European Commission (Pharmacovigilance: Overview).

Regulators are increasingly relying on RWE to inform decision-making on drug product safety profiles, especially via observational studies. Such studies are considered non-randomized, non-interventional studies; in other words, these are studies where an investigator observes individuals without intervention or manipulation. This is in contrast to randomized controlled trials where investigators observe the specific effects of a particular intervention on a pre-determined outcome.

In the US, according to the FDA's 2018 "Framework for FDA's RWE Program" (Real-World Evidence Program, US FDA 2018), there are already significant uses of RWE for the purposes of monitoring and evaluating safety of a drug, following its initial approval, i.e., in the post-marketing setting. RWD (e.g., medical claims and pharmacy dispensing data) can be considered the FDA's primary source for performing pharmacoepidemiologic queries and studies, with such data derived from the Sentinel System, as described below.

The Sentinel System Initiative is an infrastructure launched in May 2008 by the Department of Health and Human Service (HHS) to support the Sentinel System and FDA-Catalyst. The Sentinel System was designed to complement existing FDA surveillance capabilities that track AE- reports to further inform medical product safety and allow the Agency to proactively assess the safety of marketed products (About the Food and Drug Administration (FDA) Sentinel Initiative). Currently, the Sentinel System contains data on more than 100 million individuals and exists within a network of 24 collaborating institutions and 16 data partners contributing data to the model (FDA's Sentinel program). FDA uses multiple data sources to analyse drug and biologic utilization in the market to evaluate if any new safety issues or signals arise that require regulatory action or issuance of a query to the sponsor. The FDA-Catalyst is a platform within the Sentinel infrastructure designed to answer a wide range of questions by supplementing data from the Sentinel System with information from insurance plan members and providers. The Harvard Pilgrim Health Care Institute, as leader of the Sentinel System Coordinating Center, partners with data and academic partners to provide healthcare data and scientific, technical, and organizational expertise for purposes of addressing FDA questions. These partners are defined as Collaborating Institutions.

Other relevant initiatives have been developed within the Sentinel System to focus surveillance on specific medicines e.g., Post-Licensure Market Rapid Immunization Safety Monitoring (PRISM) system for vaccine safety and Sentinel Biologics Effectiveness and Safety (BEST) system for biologic medicines.

The utility of RWE for purposes of further characterizing the safety profile of a product in a post-market setting can be extremely valuable. As an example, using RWD derived from the Sentinel System, the FDA indicated they were able to provide an efficient and accurate post-market evaluation on nine potential safety issues involving five drug products. This ultimately had two major benefits: (1) eliminating the need for product sponsors to design and conduct controlled post-marketing studies, which are expensive and take years to complete, and (2) allowing for a more timely evaluation of potential safety issues, thus the ability to provide important information to patients and healthcare prescribers. Pharmaceutical companies can leverage similar techniques to answer important safety questions about their therapies and build a case to support recommendations to regulatory bodies, patients and prescribers, based on RWD.

Regardless of the potential advantages of harnessing RWE for the purpose of further characterizing the safety of a product, there are some limitations. Such limitations primarily include bias introduced by the inconsistency in the nature of the data sourced and confounding i.e., variables that can influence the dependent and independent variables being measured thus skewing the results. Such limitations can be mitigated by properly-designed and well-discussed protocol and statistical analysis plan with the health authority of interest or other statistical or non-statistical strategies (Beaulieu-Jones et al., 2020). Furthermore, global health authorities have specific programs or pilot programs designed to help assess utility of RWE and other novel approaches to reach a common goal, like drug safety characterization. As expressed in this chapter, FDA and other regulators are willing to think creatively and collaborate with industry in the interest of public health to ensure the safety and effectiveness of drugs.

In the context of post-marketing safety surveillance, leveraging modern technology and analytics to generate RWE can significantly reduce sponsor time and monetary resources to address expectations of health authorities and other stakeholders and do so with greater efficiency (e.g., payers, healthcare decision makers, etc.). RWE can serve as a beneficial tool in post-marketing safety surveillance and may support modernization of regulatory decision-making paradigm while maintaining high evidence standards. RWD and RWE can allow regulators and sponsors to identify and track a wide range of safety signals, thus enabling faster communication to regulatory authorities, patients and healthcare prescribers.

2.3 Clinical Trial Optimization

Aside from the post-marketing space, RWE can offer benefits in all stages of the clinical development spectrum (Bipartisan Policy Centre 2016). Specifically, RWE can help optimize and enrich RCT designs and can prove useful across all phases of drug development, including preclinical, clinical trial design and implementation, and post-approval commitments in pharmacovigilance and safety. There are several areas that RWE can provide trial feasibility and hypothesis-generalization information (Figure 2.2).

The drug development process typically relies on clinical trials (Figure 2.1, Table 2.1). According to the U.S. FDA (2020a), 'clinical trials' are defined

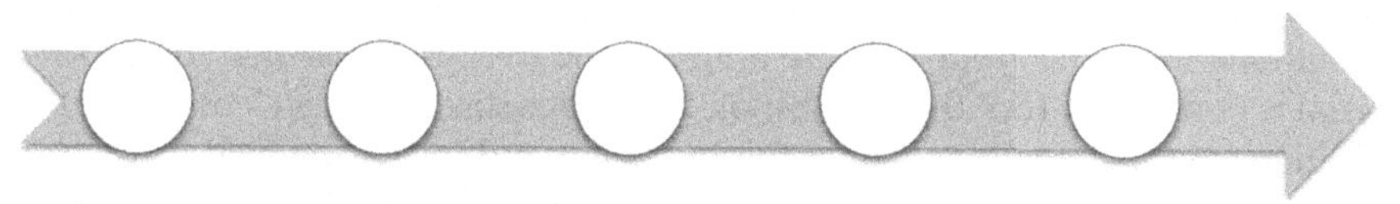

FIGURE 2.1
Five steps in the process (FDA, 2020b).

TABLE 2.1

Four Phases of Randomized Controlled Trials

Phase	Purpose	Patient Sample Size	Duration	Proportion Drugs Moving onto Next Phase
1	Safety and dosage	20 to 100 healthy volunteers or people with the disease/condition	Several months	70%
2	Efficacy and side effects	Up to several hundred people with the disease/condition	Several months to 2 years	33%
3	Efficacy and monitoring of adverse reactions	300 to 3,000 volunteers who have the disease or condition	1 to 4 years	25–30%
4	Safety and efficacy	Several thousand volunteers who have the disease/condition	Not Specified	Not Applicable

Source: FDA (2020b).

as: "voluntary research studies conducted in people and designed to answer specific questions about the safety or effectiveness of drugs, vaccines, other therapies, or new ways of using existing treatments."

For well over 50 years randomized controlled trials (RCTs) have been considered the "gold standard" to prove drug efficacy and confirm positive benefit risk ratio for intended use in a specified population or multiple populationss. Whilst RCTs provide robust efficacy and safety information about a drug, these data are classically generated under ideal and strictly controlled conditions not representative of real-world clinical practice settings. RCTs can therefore have certain limitations such as lack of or low representation of patients with multiple comorbidities or coadministration with other drugs, unrepresented age groups, races, gender or ethnicities, and possible limitations in ability to detect rare and chronic toxicities that may occur once a trial is concluded (Booth and Tannok 2014, Bipartisan Policy Centre 2016). In addition, in the new age of precision medicine and individualized care, RCTs will likely fall short in generating adequate data where variability in genetics, environment, and lifestyle require drugs and diagnostics tailored to treat very specific subsets of patients (Bipartisan Policy Centre 2016). Generating clinical data from traditional RCTs can be challenging in rare diseases, or from pediatric patients; where patient populations may be small, geographically scattered, difficult to recruit or pose ethical challenges and are therefore problematic to access (Safe and Effective Medicines for Children, Chiaruttini, Felisi and Bonifazi 2018).

RWE can inform and refine design of clinical study protocols by providing sponsors with insight into meaningful endpoints to measure for purposes of hypothesis generation. RWD, such as patient registries, can also provide sponsors insight into patient needs and help identify the population or populations who might benefit from a particular therapy; as such, recruitment of the right subjects into a trial translates into a more informed study potentially reducing the amount of data needed to demonstrate a treatment effect e.g. sample size optimization (Bipartisan Policy Centre 2016). The various ways in which RWE and RWD can be leveraged to optimize clinical trials are described in Figures 2.2–2.4.

It is imperative to identify methods to optimize diversity in clinical trials to ensure generalizeability; diversity in clinical trials is a high priority initiaive for many health authorities and pharmaceutical companies. According to the FDA's (2020e) guidance, "consider using real-world data to promote more efficient recruitment of a diverse population by using, for example, claims data and electronic health records (while maintaining patient privacy and ensuring that patient permissions/consent for the sharing/access of identifiable data from electronic health records is obtained and maintained) to identify potential sites and participants."

As an example of how RWD is being used in the setting of COVID-19, in the Reagan-Udall Foundation's (2020) and FDA's (2020d) COVID-19 Evidence Accelerator, the performance of diagnostic and antibody tests will be examined using RWD, as well as testing strategies to evaluate the prevalence of disease, chains of transmission, and individual and population-level immunity.

In another example of a general approach using RWD, an assessment of variables examined through RWD (Table 2.2) allowed for optimization of a Phase 2 RCT after identifying a bottleneck of slow enrollment due to rigorous inclusion and exclusion criteria.

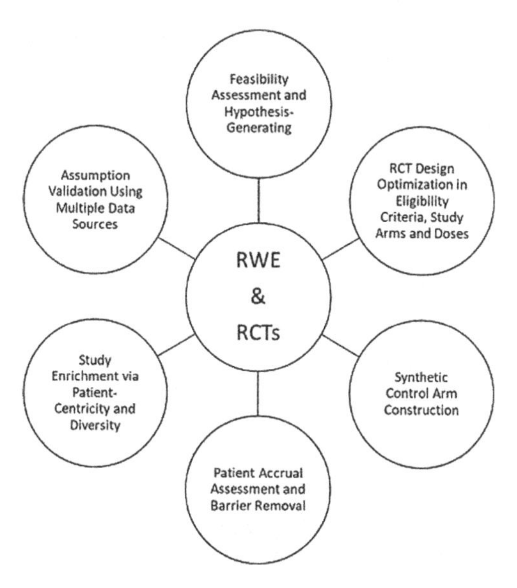

FIGURE 2.2
The roles of RWE in RCTs.

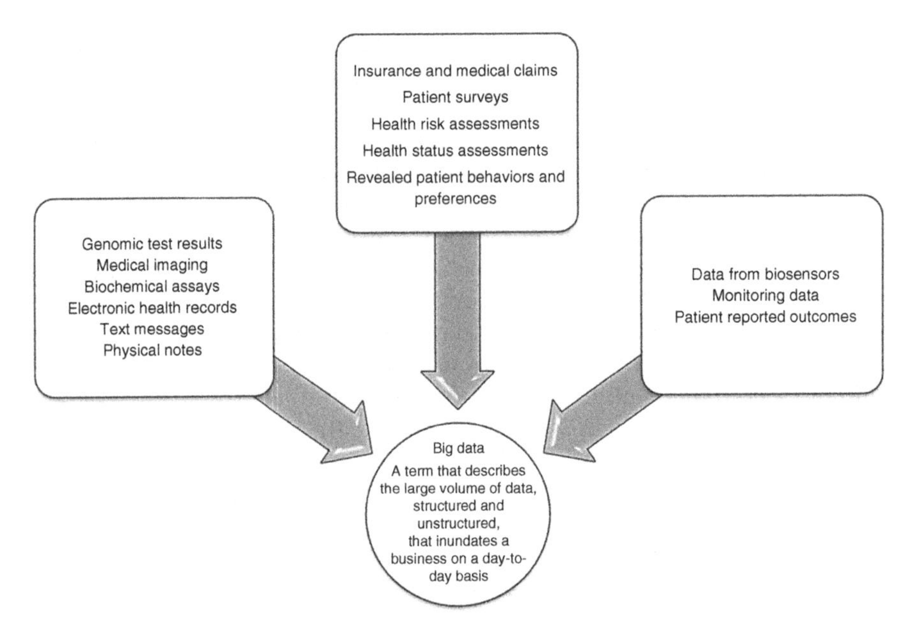

FIGURE 2.3
The role of big data that can be leveraged to optimize RCTs.

TABLE 2.2

Statistical Variables Commonly Available From Real-World Databases

Category	Patient Demographics & Socioeconomics	Participant Reported Outcomes/Clinical Data	Treatments Resource Use/Cost
Statistical Variables	Age, sex, region, payer, region Height/weight (but may not be as accurate)	Current/recent medication use (including over-the-counter (OTC)) Knowledge and health beliefs	Out-of-pocket expenses
	Life-style changes Risk factors: alcohol use, smoking history, family history Socioeconomic status (education, income, etc.)	Patients' reported compliance/adherence to treatments Quality of life Satisfaction with treatment Self-reported disease diagnoses/ symptoms/ progression Work productivity	Recent healthcare resource use (lab tests, visits to physician offices, hospital admission, prescriptions, etc.)

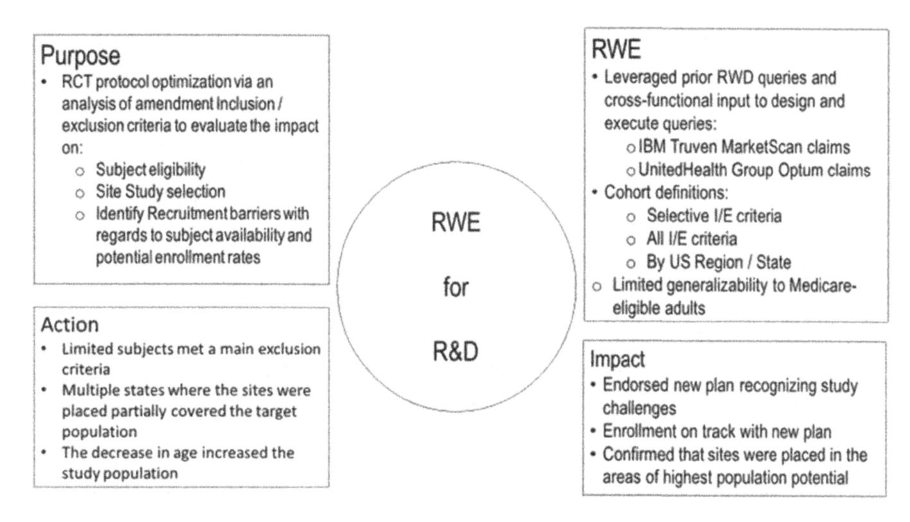

FIGURE 2.4
RCT-optimization of a Phase 2 trial.

2.4 RWE for HTA Purposes

Despite current and potential uses discussed thus far for RWE and RWD, RWD requirements for health technology assessment (HTA) purposes are varied. There are some available tools that can be employed to support this application, such as E2C (i.e., "evidence to claim"), observational HEOR studies, budget impact analysis (U.S. Department of Veterans Affairs, 2020), and risk-sharing value-based contracts (U.S. National Pharmaceutical Council, 2020) to demonstrate product differentiation, adoption, and switch patterns. Across different HTA agencies in the EU, policies for RWD use exist around pharmacoeconomic analysis, drug reimbursement discussions, and conditional drug reimbursement schemes; however, such policies differ among these contexts and could discourage use of RWD for HTA Makady et al. (2017).

Makady et al. (2017) summarized the receptiveness of RWE by different HTA bodies. The key takeaway is that differences emerged between agencies' use and recommendations for RWD use depending on the context; no visible trends for RWD use over time were observed.

1. England [National Institute for Health and Care Excellence (NICE)]
2. Scotland [Scottish Medicines Consortium (SMC)]
3. France [Haute Autorité de santé (HAS)]
4. Germany [Institute for Quality and Efficacy in Healthcare (IQWiG)]
5. The Netherlands [Zorginstituut Nederland (ZIN)]

Angelis et al. (2018) compared the following HTA agencies with respect to their practices, processes and policies of value-assessment for new medicines. Of note, various countries evaluated a similar set of evidence but methodology across the agencies varied. For example, the 'accepable data sources' for consideration in the HTA varied across agencies – some allowing for consideration of observational data (e.g. RWE, RWD) and others not.

1. France (Haute Autorité de Santé, HAS)
2. Germany (Institut für Qualität und Wirtschaftlichkeit im Gesundheitswesen, IQWiG)
3. Sweden (Tandvårds- och läkemedelsförmånsverket, TLV)
4. England (National Institute for Health and Care Excellence, NICE)
5. Italy (Agenzia Italiana del Farmaco, AIFA)
6. The Netherlands [Zorginstituut Nederland, ZIN (formerly College voor zorgverzekeringen, CVZ)]
7. Poland (The Agency for Health Technology Assessment and Tariff System, AOTMiT)
8. Spain [Red de Agencias de Evaluación de Tecnologías Sanitarias y Prestaciones del Sistema Nacional de Salud (RedETS) and the Interministerial Committee for Pricing (ICP)].

Thus, regulatory authorities and pharmaceutical companies need to focus on collaboration and partnering in policy development to harmonize methodologies related to HTAs.

2.5 Label Expansion & Drug Approvals

Label expansion initiatives for approved drugs, such as the addition of a new indication or extending an approved indication to include new patient groups, typically require additional data from adequate well-designed clinical trials. Such trials must confirm that the drug can safely and effectively treat the patient populations other than those for which it was originally intended (Novel Approach Allows Expansion of Indication for Cystic Fibrosis Drug, US FDA, Development & Approval Process -Drugs, US FDA).

RWE can provide a valuable source of data to support label expansion for already approved drugs in areas such as modification or inclusion of new indications, change in doses and dosing regimens or route of administration (Framework for FDA's Real-World Evidence Program), to add comparative effectiveness information or safety information (FDA's Guidance for Industry) and for the expansion of indications to broaden patient populations, e.g.; inclusion of pediatric populations for a product indication initially approved in adults (Franklin et al., 2019). RWE can provide important insights about drug usage and potential barriers to such use, revealing useful information about efficacy and safety of drugs used in a real-world medical practice setting (Gajra et al., 2020).

Health authorities globally are increasingly accepting of the use of RWE to support label expansion initiatives and recognize this can be particularly valuable to inform regulatory decision making as discussed in the following examples. (Safe and Effective Medicines for Children, Chiaruttini, Felisi and Bonifazi. 2018).

In April 2019 Health Canada relied on evidence generated from real-world data from the National Ambulatory Medical Care Survey and National Hospital Ambulatory Medical Care Survey to approve label expansion for an already registered pediatric indication for Prevnar 13 to include active immunization for the prevention of acute otitis media in infants and children from 6 weeks to 5 years of age (Baumfeld et. al, 2020, Prevnar® 13 (Pneumococcal 13-valent Conjugate Vaccine) Product Monograph).

Another example is demonstrated by the US FDA and EMA approval of Amgen Inc.'s BLINCYTO® for the treatment of a type of leukemia (B-cell precursor acute lymphoblastic leukemia: "ALL") in patients who are in remission but have a certain risk factor for relapse (FDA expands approval of BLINCYTO® for treatment of a type of leukemia in patients who have a certain risk factor for relapse, Real-world Evidence – From Safety to a Potential Tool for Advancing Innovative Ways to Develop New Medical Therapies). The approval was based on a single-arm clinical trial that included 86 patients based on evidence of complete remission (CR) and duration of CR from a single-arm trial, the response rate of which was compared to historical data from a population of patients not treated with the drug at several U.S. and European clinical centers. Confirmatory phase 3 studies a few years later established full approval for this expanded indication (Framework for FDA's Real-World Evidence Program, US FDA 2018, Real-world Evidence – From Safety to a Potential Tool for Advancing Innovative Ways to Develop New Medical Therapies, FDA expands approval of Blincyto for treatment of a type of leukemia in patients who have a certain risk factor for relapse, European Commission Approves BLINCYTO® (blinatumomab) in Patients With Philadelphia Chromosome Negative Minimal Residual Disease-Positive B-cell Precursor Acute Lymphoblastic Leukemia).

In 2015 Pfizer's IBRANCE® (palbociclib) was initially approved for the treatment of female breast cancer and later received US FDA approval in an extremely short time frame (Morgan et al., 2020) to expand indications in combination with an aromatase inhibitor or fulvestrant to include men with hormone receptor-positive (HR+), human epidermal growth factor receptor 2-negative (HER2-) advanced or metastatic breast cancer (Morgan et al., 2020). "The approval was based on data from electronic health records and post marketing reports of the real-world use of Ibrance in male patients sourced from three databases: IQVIA Insurance database, Flatiron Health Breast Cancer database and the Pfizer global safety database" (U.S. FDA Approves IBRANCE® (palbociclib) for the Treatment of Men with HR+, HER2- Metastatic Breast Cancer).

Aside from label expansion, there have been, on occasion, utilization of RWE to support full approval of a new therapy. This is evidenced by the US FDA approval of BRINEURA® for a rare pediatric neurologic disease leading to early death (Real-world Evidence – From Safety to a Potential Tool for Advancing Innovative Ways to Develop New Medical Therapies, FDA approves first treatment for a form of Batten disease, US FDA). The efficacy of BRINEURA® was established in a non-randomized, single-arm dose escalation clinical study in 22 symptomatic pediatric patients with CLN2 (neuronal ceroid lipofuscinosis type 2) disease and compared to 42 untreated patients with CLN2 disease from a natural history disease registry (an independent historical control group) (Real-world Evidence – From Safety to a Potential Tool for Advancing Innovative Ways to Develop New Medical Therapies, FDA approves first treatment for a form of Batten disease, US FDA). This scenario demonsrates that registries can provide a beneficial and potentially high-quality source of RWD and can capture clinical outcomes of a defined patient population.

Depending on the nature of the disease and feasibility of carrying out additional clinical research, RWE can reduce or, in some cases, eliminate the need for sponsors to conduct additional lengthy, expensive trials before they can make a medicine available to patients in need.

In some cases, a medicine might be used off-label in a real-world setting at the discretion of a physician (i.e. in a population not approved for use). These data are shared with pharmaceutical companies through post-marketing surveillance; exploration of data from such experiences can help assessments on the potential benefits and risks of a particular medicine in a new population for which it is not currently indicated (Bipartisan Policy Centre 2016).

2.6 Health Authority Perspectives

In the United States, the 21st Century Cures Act intends to accelerate medical product development and bring new innovations and advances faster and more efficiently to patients (Framework for FDA's Real-World Evidence Program, US FDA).

> Section 3022 of this Cures Act requires FDA to establish a program to evaluate the potential use of RWE to help to support the approval of a new indication for a drug approved under section 505(c) of the Federal Food, Drug, and Cosmetic Act (FD&C Act) and to help to support or satisfy post approval study requirements.
>
> *Submitting Documents Using Real-World Data and Real-World Evidence to FDA for Drugs and Biologics*

The FDA thus created a framework (Figure 2.5) to evaluate the potential use of RWE to support regulatory decision making (Sherman et al., 2016, Framework for FDA's Real-World Evidence Program, US FDA). The FDA's RWE program also covers biological products and considers sources of RWE to include data from hybrid or pragmatic trial designs and observational studies that could potentially be used to evaluate label expansion or changes pertaining to product effectiveness, including the following: adding or modifying of indications, changes in dose, dose regimen, or route of administration; adding a new population; adding comparative effectiveness or safety information (Framework for FDA's Real-World Evidence Program, US FDA, FDA's Sentinel Initiative, US FDA). RWD and RWE can also play an important role in analyzing disease burden to inform diversity plans for RCTs, therefore optimizing inclusion of underrepresented populations in clinical research (FDA, 2022).

The EMA and heads of the national competent authorities in the European Economic Area (EEA), referred to as the Heads of Medicines Agencies (HMA), established the HMA–EMA Joint Big Data task force composed

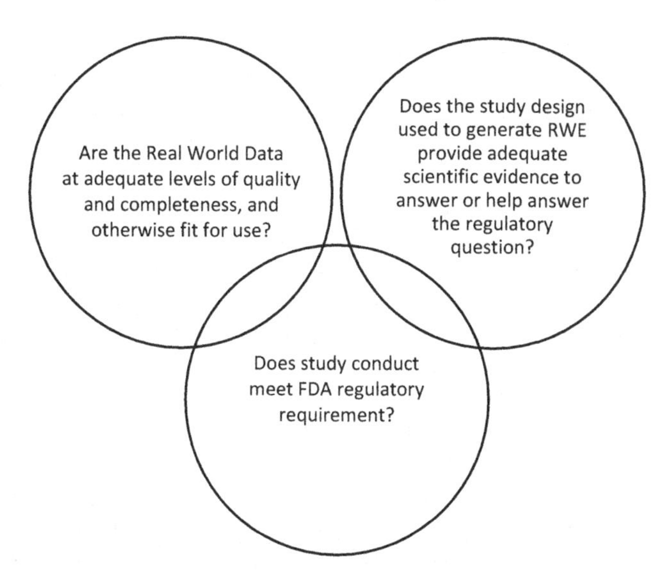

FIGURE 2.5
FDA Framework to evaluate RWD/RWE in Regulatory Decision-Making (Framework for FDA's Real-World Evidence Program, US FDA).

of representatives from 14 National Competent Authorities (NCAs) plus EMA representation, with the intent to define "big data" from a regulatory perspective and ensure the EU regulatory system holds the capability and capacity to guide, analyze and interpret these data (EMA/105321/2019) and "to explore how medicines regulators in the EEA can use big data to support research, innovation and robust medicines development in order to benefit human and animal health" (EMA/189364/2017). The HMA-EMA task force applies the following definition to big data;

> extremely large datasets which may be complex, multi-dimensional, unstructured and heterogeneous, which are accumulating rapidly and which may be analyzed computationally to reveal patterns, trends, and associations. In general, big data sets require advanced or specialized methods to provide an answer within reliable constraints.

The task force issued an Interim Summary Report in February 2019, with recommendations for a path towards understanding the acceptability of evidence derived from "big data" in support of the evaluation and supervision of medicines by regulators (EMA/105321/2019). In preparing the report, it assessed the generation of "big data," their relevant sources and main formats, the methods for processing and analyzing big data and the current state of expertise across the European medicines regulatory network. Six subgroups of data sources relevant to regulatory decision-making were considered by the task force: genomics, bioanalytical "omics" (proteomics, etc.), clinical trials, observational data, spontaneous adverse drug reactions data and social media and mobile health data. Final Report, "Evolving Data-Driven Regulation," issued in January 2021, provides practical recommendations on how big data could be used in support of innovation and public health. This includes 10 priority recommendations including establishing DARWIN network (HMA-EMA Joint Big Data Taskforce Phase II report, Priority Recommendations of the HMA-EMA joint Big Data Task Force). In September 2020, the EMA issued draft guidelines on registry-based studies to provide recommendations on key methodological aspects that are specific to the use of patient registries by marketing authorization applicants and holders (MAAs/MAHs) planning to conduct studies (EMA/502388/2020, Baumfeld et al., 2020). The guideline focuses on studies based on disease registries or condition registries to study the utilization, safety and effectiveness of medicines prescribed to or consumed by patients included in the registry and provides examples where registry-based studies may be useful for evidence generation which includes provision of data sources or infrastructure for post-authorization evidence generation which in the context of products that have been previously investigated in RCTs, registry-based studies may help, for example, to estimate and predict the effectiveness of adapted drug dosing schemes applied in clinical practice and understand effectiveness and safety of medicinal products in a broader clinical disease-related context and a more heterogenous patient population (EMA/502388/2020).

The EMA also introduced the "Adaptive Pathways" approach, which is based on the scientific concept for medicine development and data generation to enable early and progressive patient access to a medicine. Whilst the standards and requirements to confirm positive benefits risk ratios within the existing EU regulatory framework for medicines will continue, the adaptive pathway is built upon three principles which include: gathering evidence through real-life use (e.g., RWD) as a supplement to clinical trial data, iterative development, meaning approval in stages which begins with restricted patient populations and extends to broader patient populations or confirmation of a products positive benefit-risk following conditional approval based on early data, and early participation of patients and HTA bodies in a medicine's development process.

In Canada, Health Canada continues to encourage sponsors on the use of RWE to support regulatory submissions and in 2019 publicly announced ongoing initiatives to optimize use of RWE for regulatory decisions to improve the extent and rate of access to prescription drugs in Canada highlighting key partnerships with organizations, including the Canadian Agency for Drugs and Technologies in Health (CADTH), the Institut national d'excellence en santé et en services sociaux (INESSS) and collaborations with HTA organizations to establish a joint document that will optimize and formalize the use of RWE during the drug product life cycle (Optimizing the Use of Real-world Evidence to Inform Regulatory Decision-Making, Government of Canada). They additionally released a document entitled "Elements of Real-world Data/Evidence Quality throughout the Prescription Drug Product Life Cycle" to provide an outline and guidance on protocol elements and data quality considerations during the data collection and evaluation of RWE with intent to update the document with the evolving expertise and experience in this area (Optimizing the Use of Real-world Evidence to Inform Regulatory Decision-Making, Government of Canada).

In January 2020, the National Medical Products Administration (NMPA) of China released interim Guidelines for RWE to Support Drug Development and Review providing guidance and standardization on the use of RWE in drug R&D and review.

The PMDA of Japan has been utilizing RWD to assess drug safety since 2009 and have more recently updated regulatory guidelines, which promote RWD utilization by pharmaceutical industries in pharmacovigilance. The PMDA describes challenges in utilizing RWD for regulatory in areas of "data quality, data coding, deep understanding about databases, validation of clinical outcomes and system infrastructure, and timely and continuous communication with marketing authorization holders (MAH)" (Uyama 2018, Ando. T). The PMDA have acknowledged the need for international cooperation with regulatory agencies and stakeholders to share information and experiences to enable movement to international harmonization efforts in utilizing RWD in the regulatory process; a position other agencies such as the US FDA and EMA have similarly expressed in their guidance documents on the subject, for example; Framework For FDA's Real-world Evidence Program and HMA/EMA Joint Task Force Summary Report respectively (Ando. T, EMA/105321/2019, Framework for FDA's Real-World Evidence Program, US FDA).

The increasing prevalence and acceptance of RWD and RWE to inform regulatory decision making by regulators globally, particularly major health authorities like the FDA and EMA, supports the notion that effectively harnessing the copious volumes of available health data from EHRs, claims databases, electronic devices, software applications clinical practice registries, and social media will not only benefit pharmaceutical companies, but more importantly - patients. Sources of RWD can provide new and valuable insights into states of health and illness and can potentially support getting medicines in the hands of patients faster. Utilization in the setting of drug effectiveness and new drug approvals, apart from certain unique cases, is still limited. This presents opportunities for the evolution of new methodologies that can generate RWE with adequate scientific rigor to support such regulatory assesments (FDA's Sentinel Initiative, US FDA, Sentinel Initiative, Baumfeld et al., 2020). Finally, whilst there is still much work to be undertaken in RWD/RWE data organization/collection, data privacy/protection, and verification of data quality, RWD will prove invaluable in drug development and accessibility (Sherman et al., 2016).

Disclaimer

Corinne S. Pillai, Ewa Filipowska and Kelly H. Zou are employees of Viatris, merged between Upjohn, a Division of Pfizer, and Mylan. Eleanor E. Panico is a former employee of Upjohn, a Division of Pfizer, and Viatris. The views expressed are the authors' own and do not necessarily represent those of their employer or employers. The authors appreciate the editorial support from Arghya Bhattacharya and Aswin Kumar A of Viatris.

References

21st Century Cures Act, US FDA 2020, Available at: www.fda.gov/regulatory-information/selected-amendments-fdc-act/21st-century-cures-act (accessed on December 19, 2021).

About the Food and Drug Administration (FDA) Sentinel Initiative, Available at: www.sentinelinitiative.org/about_us (accessed on December 19, 2021).

Ando. T., Recent Trend on Utilization of Real-world Data - Challenges in Japan, Office of Medical Informatics and Epidemiology (OME) Pharmaceuticals and Medical Devices Agency (PMDA). Available at: www.pmda.go.jp/files/000226214.pdf (accessed on December 19, 2021).
Angelis, A., Lange, A., Kanavos, P. Using health technology assessment to assess the value of new medicines: results of a systematic review and expert consultation across eight European countries. Eur J Health Econ. 2018 Jan;19(1):123–152.
Baumfeld Andre, E., Reynolds, R., Caubel, P., Azoulay, L. and Dreyer, N.A., 2020. Trial designs using real-world data: the changing landscape of the regulatory approval process. Pharmacoepidemiology and Drug Safety, 29(10), pp.1201–1212.
Beaulieu-Jones, B.K., Finlayson, S.G., Yuan, W., Altman, R.B., Kohane, I.S., Prasad, V. and Yu, K.H., 2020. Examining the use of real-world evidence in the regulatory process. Clinical Pharmacology & Therapeutics, 107(4), pp.843–852.
Berger, M.L., Sox, H., Willke, R.J., et al. Good Practices for Real-World Data Studies of Treatment and/or Comparative Effectiveness: Recommendations from the Joint ISPOR-ISPE Special Task Force on Real-World Evidence in Health Care Decision Making. Value in Health. 2017; 20(8): 1003–1008.
Booth, C.M. and Tannock, I.F., 2014. Randomised controlled trials and population-based observational research: partners in the evolution of medical evidence. British Journal of Cancer, 110(3), pp.551–555.
CFR – Code of Federal Regulations Title 21, Available at: www.accessdata.fda.gov/scripts/cdrh/cfdocs/cfcfr/CFRSearch.Cfm?fr=314.80 (accessed on December 19, 2021).
Chiaruttini, G., Felisi, M. and Bonifazi, D., 2018. Challenges in paediatric clinical trials: How to Make It Feasible. The Management of Clinical Trials. Rijeka: Intech, pp.11–33.
Committee on Pediatric Studies Conducted Under the Best Pharmaceuticals for Children Act (BPCA) and the Pediatric Research Equity Act (PREA); Board on Health Sciences Policy; Institute of Medicine; Field, M.J., Boat, T.F., editors. Safe and Effective Medicines for Children: Pediatric Studies Conducted Under the Best Pharmaceuticals for Children Act and the Pediatric Research Equity Act. Washington (DC): National Academies Press (US); 2012 Feb 29. 4, Ethical Issues in Pediatric Drug Studies. Available from: www.ncbi.nlm.nih.gov/books/NBK202037/ (accessed on December 19, 2021).
CONSORT – CONsolidated Standards Of Reporting Trials. About CONSORT. 2010.
Data Analysis and Real-world Interrogation Network (DARWIN EU), Available at: www.ema.europa.eu/en/about-us/how-we-work/big-data/data-analysis-real-world-interrogation-network-darwin-eu (accessed on December 19, 2021).
Department of Veterans Affairs. Budget Impact Analysis. 2020. www.herc.research.va.gov/include/page.asp?id=budget-impact-analysis
Development & Approval Process -Drugs, US FDA, Available at: www.fda.gov/drugs/development-approval-process-drugs (accessed on December 19, 2021).
Dreyer, N.A., Bryant, A., Velentgas, P. The GRACE Checklist: A Validated Assessment Tool for High Quality Observational Studies of Comparative Effectiveness. Journal of Managed Care and Specialty Pharmacy 2016; 22(10):1107–1013.
European Commission Approves BLINCYTO® (blinatumomab) In Patients With Philadelphia Chromosome Negative Minimal Residual Disease-Positive B-cell

Precursor Acute Lymphoblastic Leukemia, available at: www.amgen.com/newsroom/press-releases/2019/01/european-commission-approves-blincyto-blinatumomab-in-patients-with-philadelphia-chromosome-negative-minimal-residual-diseasepositive-bcell-precursor-acute-lymphoblastic-leukemia (accessed on December 19, 2021).

FDA approves first treatment for a form of Batten disease, US FDA Press release 2017, Available at: www.fda.gov/news-events/press-announcements/fda-approves-first-treatment-form-batten-disease (accessed on December 19, 2021). FDA expands approval of Blincyto for treatment of a type of leukemia in patients who have a certain risk factor for relapse, Available at: www.fda.gov/news-events/press-announcements/fda-expands-approval-blincyto-treatment-type-leukemia-patients-who-have-certain-risk-factor-relapse (accessed on December 19, 2021).

FDA's Sentinel Initiative, US FDA, Available at: www.fda.gov/safety/fdas-sentinel-initiative (accessed on December 19, 2021).

Food and Drug Administration. Clinical Trials: What Patients Need to Know. 2020a. www.fda.gov/patients/clinical-trials-what-patients-need-know

Food and Drug Administration. Step 3: Clinical Research, The Drug Development Process. 2020b. www.fda.gov/patients/drug-development-process/step-3-clinical-research (accessed on December 19, 2021).

Food & Drug Administration. Real-World Evidence. 2020c. www.fda.gov/science-research/science-and-research-special-topics/real-world-evidence (accessed on December 19, 2021).

Food & Drug Administration. Coronavirus (COVID-19) Update: FDA Takes Additional Action to Harness Real-World Data to Inform COVID-19 Response Efforts. 2020d. www.fda.gov/news-events/press-announcements/coronavirus-covid-19-update-fda-takes-additional-action-harness-real-world-data-inform-covid-19 (accessed on December 19, 2021).

Food and Drug Administration. Enhancing the Diversity of Clinical Trial Populations--Eligibility Criteria, Enrollment Practices, and Trial Designs. 2020e. www.fda.gov/news-events/press-announcements/fda-offers-guidance-enhance-diversity-clinical-trials-encourage-inclusivity-medical-product (accessed on December 19, 2021).

Food and Drug Administration. Clinical Trial Diversity. 2022. www.fda.gov/consumers/minority-health-and-health-equity/clinical-trial-diversity (accessed on May 22, 2022).

Framework for FDA's Real-World Evidence Program, US FDA 2018, Available at: www.fda.gov/media/120060/download (accessed on December 19, 2021).

Framework for FDA's Real-World Evidence Program, US FDA, Available at: www.fda.gov/media/120060/download (accessed on December 19, 2021).

Franklin, J.M., Glynn, R.J., Martin, D. and Schneeweiss, S. 2019. Evaluating the use of nonrandomized real-world data analyses for regulatory decision making. Clinical Pharmacology & Therapeutics, 105(4), pp.867–877.

Gajra A, Zettler ME, Feinberg BA. Randomization versus Real-World Evidence. N Engl J Med. 2020 Jul 23;383(4):e21

Gamerman, V., Cai, T., Elsäßer, A. Pragmatic randomized clinical trials: best practices and statistical guidance. Health Services and Outcomes Research Methodology 2019; 19: 23–35.

Good Pharmacovigilance Practices and Pharmacoepidemiologic Assessment, US FDA 2015, Available at: www.fda.gov/regulatory-information/search-fda-guidance-documents/good-pharmacovigilance-practices-and-pharmacoepidemiologic-assessment (accessed on December 19, 2021). GRACE. Good Research for Comparative Effectiveness. 2021.

Guideline on registry-based studies, EMA/502388/2020, Available at: www.ema.europa.eu/en/documents/scientific-guideline/guideline-registry-based-studies_en.pdf (accessed on December 19, 2021).

HMA-EMA Joint Big Data Taskforce Phase II report: 'Evolving Data-Driven Regulation', Available at: www.ema.europa.eu/en/documents/other/hma-ema-joint-big-data-taskforce-phase-ii-report-evolving-data-driven-regulation_en.pdf (accessed on December 19, 2021).35.

HMA-EMA Joint Big Data Taskforce Summary report, EMA/105321/2019, Available at: www.ema.europa.eu/en/documents/minutes/hma/ema-joint-task-force-big-data-summary-report_en.pdf (accessed on December 19, 2021).36.

Katkade, V.B., Sanders, K.N., Zou, K.H. Real-world data: an opportunity to supplement existing evidence for the use of long-established medicines in health care decision making. J Multidiscip Healthc. 2018 Jul 2;11:295–304.

Makady, A., van Veelen, A., Jonsson, P., Moseley, O., D'Andon, A., de Boer, A., Hillege, H., Klungel, O., Goettsch, W. Using Real-World Data in Health Technology Assessment (HTA) Practice: A Comparative Study of Five HTA Agencies. Pharmacoeconomics. 2018 Mar; 36(3):359–368.

Morgan, J., Feghali, K., Shah, S., Miranda, W. RWE focus is shifting to R&D, early investments begin to pay off. 2020. www2.deloitte.com/us/en/insights/industry/health-care/real-world-evidence-study.html?id=us:2sm:3li:4di_gl:5eng:6di (accessed on December 19, 2021).

Morgan, J., Feghali, K., Shah, S., Miranda, W., RWE focus is shifting to R&D, early investments begin to pay off, Deloitte Insights, 2020, Available at: www2.deloitte.com/us/en/insights/industry/health-care/real-world-evidence-study.html?id=us:2sm:3li:4di_gl:5eng:6di#endnote-13 (accessed on December 19, 2021).

National Pharmaceutical Council. Value-Based Contracts. 2020. www.npcnow.org/issues/access/provider-reimbursement/risk-sharing-agreements (accessed on December 19, 2021).

Novel Approach Allows Expansion of Indication for Cystic Fibrosis Drug, US FDA, Available at: www.fda.gov/drugs/news-events-human-drugs/novel-approach-allows-expansion-indication-cystic-fibrosis-drug (accessed on December 19, 2021).

Optimizing the Use of Real World Evidence to Inform Regulatory Decision-Making, Government of Canada, Available at: www.canada.ca/en/health-canada/services/drugs-health-products/drug-products/announcements/optimizing-real-world-evidence-regulatory-decisions.html (accessed on December 19, 2021).

Pharmacovigilance: Overview, Available at: www.ema.europa.eu/en/human-regulatory/overview/pharmacovigilance-overview (accessed on December 19, 2021).

Postmarketing reporting of adverse drug experiences, eCFR, Available at: https://ecfr.io/cgi-bin/text-idx?SID=fd77b7d0c2c7e0ae8925af03a2f16443&mc=true&node=se21.5.314_180&rgn=div8 (accessed on December 19, 2021).

Prevnar® 13 (Pneumococcal 13-valent Conjugate Vaccine) Product Monograph, Pfizer Canada 2019, Available at: www.pfizer.ca/sites/default/files/201908/Prevnar13-PM_E_219617_08Aug2019.pdf (accessed on December 19, 2021).

Priority Recommendations of the HMA-EMA joint Big Data Task Force, Available at: www.ema.europa.eu/en/documents/other/priority-recommendations-hma-ema-joint-big-data-task-force_en.pdf (accessed on December 19, 2021).

Questions and Answers on FDA's Adverse Event Reporting System (FAERS), Available at: www.fda.gov/drugs/surveillance/questions-and-answers-fdas-adverse-event-reporting-system-faers (accessed on December 19, 2021).

Reagan-Udall Foundation for the Food and Drug Administration and Friends of Cancer Research. COVID-19 Evidence Accelerator. 2020. https://evidenceaccelerator.org (accessed on December 19, 2021).

Real World Evidence – From Safety to a Potential Tool for Advancing Innovative Ways to Develop New Medical Therapies, Available at: www.fda.gov/drugs/news-events-human-drugs/real-world-evidence-safety-potential-tool-advancing-innovative-ways-develop-new-medical-therapies (accessed on December 19, 2021).

Sentinel Initiative, www.sentinelinitiative.org/ (accessed on December 19, 2021).

Sutter, S. Real-Word Evidence Generation System Will Be a Priority For Califf As FDA Commissioner. 2021. https://pink.pharmaintelligence.informa.com/PS145392/Real-Word-Evidence-Generation-System-Will-Be-A-Priority-For-Califf-As-FDA-Commissioner, (accessed on December 19, 2021).

Sherman, R.E., Anderson, S.A., Dal Pan, G.J., Gray, G.W., Gross, T., Hunter, N.L., LaVange, L., Marinac-Dabic, D., Marks, P.W., Robb, M.A. and Shuren, J., 2016. Real-world evidence—what is it and what can it tell us. N Engl J Med, 375(23), pp.2293–2297.

Statement from FDA Commissioner Scott Gottlieb, M.D., on FDA's new strategic framework to advance use of real-world evidence to support development of drugs and biologics, Available at: www.fda.gov/news-events/press-announcements/statement-fda-commissioner-scott-gottlieb-md-fdas-new-strategic-framework-advance-use-real-world (accessed on December 19, 2021).

Submitting Documents Using Real-World Data and Real-World Evidence to FDA for Drugs and Biologics Guidance for Industry, Available at: www.fda.gov/media/124795/download (accessed on December 19, 2021).

U.S. FDA Approves IBRANCE® (palbociclib) for the Treatment of Men with HR+ , HER2- Metastatic Breast Cancer, Available at: www.pfizer.com/news/press-release/press-release-detail/u_s_fda_approves_ibrance_palbociclib_for_the_treatment_of_men_with_hr_her2_metastatic_breast_cancer (accessed on December 19, 2021).

Use of big data to improve human and animal health, EMA/189364/2017, Available at: www.ema.europa.eu/en/news/use-big-data-improve-human-animal-health (accessed on December 19, 2021).

Using Real-World Evidence to Accelerate Safe and Effective Cures Advancing Medical Innovation for a Healthier America June 2016, Bipartisan Policy Centre, Available at: https://bipartisanpolicy.org/download/?file=/wp-content/uploads/2019/03/BPC-Health-Innovation-Safe-Effective-Cures.pdf (accessed on December 19, 2021).

Uyama. Y., Utilizing Real World Data: A PMDA Perspective, Proceedings: DIA 2018 Global Annual Meeting, Available at: https://globalforum.diaglobal.org/issue/august-2018/utilizing-real-world-data-a-pmda-perspective/ (accessed on December 19, 2021).

Velentgas, P., Dreyer, N.A., Nourjah, P., Smith, S.R., Torchia, M.M., eds. Developing a Protocol for Observational Comparative Effectiveness Research: A User's Guide. AHRQ Publication No. 12(13)-EHC099. Rockville, MD: Agency for Healthcare Research and Quality.

Wang, S.V., Pinheiro, S., Hua, W., Arlett, P., Uyama, Y., Berlin, J.A., Bartels, D.B., Kahler, K.H., Bessette, L.G., Schneeweiss, S. STaRT-RWE: structured template for planning and reporting on the implementation of real world evidence studies. BMJ. 2021 Jan 12;372:m4856.

Weidman, J.R., Belsky, K. Estimating the probability of regulatory registration success. RAPS.org. February, 2020. www.raps.org/news-and-articles/news-articles/2020/2/estimating-the-probability-of-regulatory-registrat (accessed on December 19, 2021).

What is an observational study? Available at: www.mrcctu.ucl.ac.uk/patients-public/about-clinical-trials/what-is-an-observational-study/, accessed on 19 December 2021

What is Pharmacovigilance? WHO, Available at: www.who.int/teams/regulation-prequalification/pharmacovigilance (accessed on December 19, 2021).

White, H., Sabarwal, S., de Hoop, T. (2014). Randomized Controlled Trials (RCTs): Methodological Briefs – Impact Evaluation No. 7, Methodological Briefs no. 7. 2014

Who Is Involved? FDA Sentinel program, Available at: www.sentinelinitiative.org/about/who-involved (accessed on December 19, 2021).

World Health Organization. (2002). The importance of pharmacovigilance. World Health Organization. https://apps.who.int/iris/handle/10665/42493 (accessed on December 19, 2021).

Zhou, S. and Johnson, R. Pharmaceutical probability of success. Alacrita Consulting. April 2019. https://cdn2.hubspot.net/hubfs/3828687/Alacrita_April2019/PDF/Pharmaceutical-Probability-of-Success.pdf (accessed on December 19, 2021).

Zou, K.H., Li, J.Z., Imperato, J., Potkar, C.N., et al. Harnessing Real-World Data for Regulatory Use and Applying Innovative Applications. J Multidiscip Healthc. 2020 Jul 22;13:671–679.

Zou, K.H., Li, J.Z., Ovalle, J. et al. Optimizing Patient Care Through AI/ML/DL. PharmaVoice. June 2020.

Zou, K.H., Li, J.Z., Salem, L.A., Imperato, J. et al. Harnessing real-world evidence to reduce the burden of noncommunicable disease: health information technology and innovation to generate insights. Health Serv Outcomes Res Methodol. 2020 Nov 6:1–13.

Zwarenstein, M., Treweek, S., Gagnier, J.J., Altman, D.G., Tunis, S., Haynes, B., Oxman, A.D., Moher, D.; CONSORT group; Pragmatic Trials in Healthcare (Practihc) group. Improving the reporting of pragmatic trials: an extension of the CONSORT statement. BMJ. 2008 Nov 11;337:a2390.

3

Patient Data Privacy, Protected Health Information, and Ethics of Real-World Evidence

Corinne S. Pillai, Eleanor E. Panico, Kelly H. Zou, and Ewa Filipowska
Viatris

CONTENTS

3.1 Data Privacy Laws

In the context of expanding utilization of and access to Real World Evidence (RWE) and Real World Data (RWD), privacy and the appropriate use of such data are of utmost importance. The United States (US) Health Insurance Portability and Accountability Act of 1996 (HIPAA 1996, Summary of HIPAA privacy rules) is a federal law enacted in August, 1996, which required the creation of national standards that would prevent the disclosure of patient

DOI: 10.1201/9781003017523-3

sensitive health data without their prior consent or knowledge. The US Department of Health and Human Services ("HHS") issued the HIPAA Privacy Rule, to allow for implementation of the requirements of HIPAA. Whilst ensuring the privacy and protection of individuals' health information, HIPAA enables the appropriate flow of this information to facilitate and support high quality healthcare (HIPAA 1996). Individuals and organizations, such as healthcare providers, health plans and healthcare clearinghouses, herein referred to as "Covered Entities" subject to the Privacy Rule, are required to abide by standards which address the use and disclosure of individuals "protected health information" or (PHI). Any individually identifiable health information held or transmitted by a covered entity or its business associate, in any form or media, whether electronic, paper, or oral is considered PHI (Summary of HIPAA privacy rules).

There are, however, certain instances where covered entities, based on professional ethics and best judgments, are permitted to use and disclose PHI, without obtaining an individual's prior authorization as depicted in Figure 3 1.

Evolving technological advancement allows the healthcare industry to steadily move from paper-based processes to use of electronic information systems. The HIPAA Security Rule protects the subset of electronic information covered by the Privacy Rule referred to as "electronic protected health

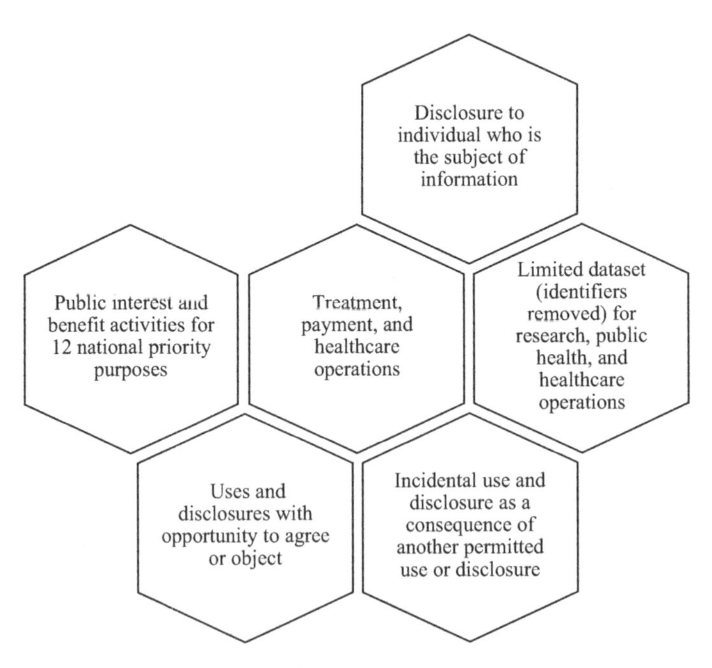

FIGURE 3.1
Permitted uses and disclosures by covered entities.

information" (e-PHI) and establishes national standards for protecting certain health information that is retained or transferred in electronic format. The Security Rule requires that covered entities ensure the confidentiality, integrity, and availability of all e-PHI; detect and safeguard against anticipated threats to the security of the information; protect against anticipated impermissible uses or disclosures and certify compliance by their workforce. The Security Rule does not apply to oral or written PHI. The Office for Civil Rights (OCR) within the HHS is responsible for the implementation and enforcement of HIPAA. Covered entities who do not voluntarily comply with the standards of the Privacy Rule may be subject to civil monetary penalties and in some instances, violations may be subject to criminal prosecution (Summary of HIPAA privacy rules).

The EU's General Data Protection Regulation (GDPR), "on the protection of natural persons with regard to the processing of personal data and on the free movement of such data", became effective in May 2018 (Fact Sheets on the European Union) and is considered one of the most stringent data privacy laws in the world. Although developed and conceded in the EU; GDPR imposes obligations on organizations anywhere in the world that collect data from individuals within the EU. The GDPR stems from the 1950 European Convention on Human Rights, which states, "Everyone has the right to respect for his private and family life, his home and his correspondence", thus the EU aims to guard this right through adequate legislation. Prior to the GDPR, The Data Protection Directive 95/46/EC4 enacted in 1995 safeguarded data privacy and the free movement of personal data within the EU states (GDPR and Anonymization, white paper, privacy analytics, REGULATION (EU) 2016/679). This original Directive, however, did not consider how technological advancements would result in prolific data creation and global scale data sharing. The GDPR replaces this original directive to account for the diverse pathways in which Personally Identifiable Information (PII) can be produced, circulated, and retrieved within a technologically charged global environment. (European data protection supervisor, GDPR and Anonymization, white paper, privacy analytics). The GDPR reinforces existing data privacy rights of EU citizens whilst also delivering new rights that allow individuals to better control and access their personal data, including the right to request deletion of personal data when no valid reason for retention exists. GDPR ensures that individuals are informed about security breaches of personal data and warrants organizations to promptly inform both individuals and data protection supervisory authorities of significant breaches. GDPR also aims to improve business innovation and advancement opportunities through unification and simplification of an EU wide regulation pertinent to organizations conducting business activities both within and outside the EU (Protection of personal data (from 2018), EurLex). Also see European Commission (2022a) and European Commission (2022b).

In Canada, the Personal Information Protection and Electronic Documents Act (PIPEDA) Act was adopted in April 2000 and applies private-sector organizations in Canada (Personal Information Protection and Electronic Documents Act.). PIPEDA intends to protect personal information collected, used, or disclosed during commercial activities and requires organizations involved in such activities to obtain an individual's consent before proceeding with any related activities that involve personal (identifiable) information. The law ensures that individuals in Canada have the right to access their personal information, contest incorrect information and understand by whom and why their information is being collected (PIPEDA).

Emerging market countries, such as China, continue to develop and improve local legislature to increase controls and standards, which regulate and protect personal information rights and standardize the flow and management of data to safeguard the rational use of personal information. Examples of key regulations in China include; Cybersecurity Law, Data Security Law, and the still-in-draft Personal Information Protection Law. The Data Security Law of the People's Republic of China, effective in September 2021 was "formulated to standardize data handling activities, ensure data security, promote data development and use and protect the lawful rights and interests of individuals and organizations, and safeguard national sovereignty, security, and development interests" (Translation: Data Security Law of the People's Republic of China, 2021). The Personal Information Protection Law of China, effective 01 November 2021, was developed on the basis of the Chinese Constitution. The Law ensures the protection of personal information rights and interests of individuals within the borders of China, and requires standardized personal information handling activities, thus promoting the rational use of personal information (Translation: Data Security Law of the People's Republic of China, 2021). The Law applies outside the borders of China when handling personal information of persons within the country's borders when "the purpose is to provide products or services to natural persons inside the borders; where analyzing or assessing activities of natural persons inside the borders or other circumstances provided in laws or administrative regulations (Translation: Data Security Law of the People's Republic of China, 2021)". The Cyber Security Law of the People's Republic of China became effective in July 2017 and was created to "safeguard cyberspace sovereignty and national security, and social and public interests; protect the lawful rights and interests of citizens, legal persons, and other organizations; and promote the healthy development of the informatization of the economy and society." Article 37 of the law states that "critical information infrastructure operators (CIIOs) who collect or generate personal information or important data during business activities within mainland China are required to store such data within mainland China". If there is a business need or rationale to share such data outside China, then CIIOs are required to conduct an applicable security assessment. Critical information infrastructure operators who fail to comply with this regulation may be subject to significant levies or fines, legal warnings, suspension of business activities, revocation of operations licenses/permits or cancellation of business licenses (Translation: Cybersecurity Law of the People's Republic of China, 2017).

As evidenced by the dynamic progression and establishment of data protection and privacy laws globally, it is apparent that governments and healthcare agencies recognize the importance of responsible utilization of personal health information and related personal data sets. A study on the "Privacy Attitudes among Early Adopters of Emerging Health Technologies"; conducted a survey which revealed that whilst individuals wanted to be "altruistic" in the sharing of their personal health data in the interests of public benefit and scientific research, they also wished to also maintain their privacy and anonymity (Cheung et al., 2016). A 2016 study report from Ipsos Mori for the Wellcome Trust titled "Public attitudes to commercial access to health data", revealed that 52% of individuals surveyed were amenable to sharing personal health data with commercial organizations for research purposes on condition that data were anonymized, whilst 17% were not willing to share personal data under any situation with reasons including a lack of trust by some respondents (20%) in commercial organizations' ability to safely store their data (IPSOS 2016, GDPR and Anonymization).

Harnessing and leveraging large volumes of health data in all its forms (e.g., structured, and unstructured) from various sources is pivotal to the progression of medical science, health technology and the evolution of drug and medical therapies. However, central to this objective is the assurance that PHI and identifiable fields are adequately protected and that individuals' rights to anonymity, autonomy and control of their personal data is appropriately preserved and respected (see, e.g., European Commission, 2022a; European Commission, 2022b).

3.2 Ethics of Real-World Evidence

Universal and industry-wide ethical and bioethical standards for real-world evidence (RWE) have not yet been well-established. In the emerging era of digital, AI and robotics; globally aligned and more consistent approaches to data integrity and patient privacy protection are even more important. Some tools have, however, been developed in the the scientific and research industry to guide internal policy/standard operating procedure development and ensure that the scientific research being pursued in this space is ethically sound (refer to Section 3.4 Best Practices). Such tools include guidance/policy documents from government bodies and best practices from professional organizations. Examples of such bodies include the United Nations, the United States (US) Food & Drug Administration (FDA), and the European Medicines Agency (EMA). Referenced below are examples of guidance that provide a foundation for ethical considerations with respect to generating and utilizing RWE.

First, the United Nations' (2020) Data Privacy, Ethics and Protection Guidance Note on Big Data for Achievement of the 2030 Agenda established common principles across UNDG to support the operational use of big data for achievement of the Sustainable Development Goals (SDGs). This guidance serves as a risk-management tool considering fundamental human rights and sets principles for obtaining, retention, use and quality control for data from the private sector.

In the US, to promote advancement in the field and to address a congressional mandate, FDA issued a series of draft guidances on various aspects of RWD and RWE in the context of regulatory decisions. Four guidances were issued in late 2021 with plans to issue additional guidance. Guidances issued thus far include the topics: (1) assessing data sources (one draft guidance on EHRs and medical claims data and one guidance on registries); (2) data standards; (3) regulatory considerations. These guidance documents discuss topics such as challenges experienced when creating a linkage between one registry to another data source to obtain supplementary information; specifically, challenges with addressing inconsistencies, protecting patient privacy, and mitigating redundant information (FDA, 2022).

European Union's (2020) General Data Protection Regulation (GDPR) is the most stringent privacy and security law in the world. Although drafted and passed by the European Union (EU), it imposes obligations on organizations anywhere in the world, if they target or collect data related to people in the EU. Compliance with GDPR becomes extremely relevant with reference to the European Medicine Agency (2020) recently developed draft guidance which emphasizes a paradigm shift from pre-approval activities to strengthened post-approval activities using RWD.

China's State Council (2016) emphasized advancing big data application in health and medical sectors to focus on building both national and provincial population health information. "National and provincial population health information platforms will be built, and application platforms for national medicine bidding and purchasing will be interconnected by the end of 2017, according to the circular." "In addition, based on current resources, 100 regional clinical medicine data demonstration centers will be built across the country."

According to KPMG's (2017) summary, China's cyber security law focuses on protecting personal information and individual privacy, as well as standardizing the collection and use of PHI. Consequently, companies must introduce data protection measures to protect sensitive data—for instance, information on Chinese citizens or relating to national security—must be stored on domestic servers. In some cases, firms will need to undergo a security review before moving data out of China. One of the challenges, however, is that the government has been unclear on what is considered important or sensitive data.

The Japanese Pharmaceutical and Medical Device Agency (PMDA, 2020), under the Medical Information Risk Assessment Initiative (MIHARI) framework, established medical information database for pharmacoepidemiological drug safety assessments known as the MID-NET® Project. It is expected that MID-NET® will become a primary source of data for clinical research and post-marketing drug safety studies conducted by the pharmaceutical industry as well as drug-safety assessments conducted by the PMDA (Yamaguchi, 2019).

The International Society for Pharmacoeconomics and Outcomes Research (ISPOR) formed a joint Special Task Force with The International Society for Pharmacoepidemiology (ISPE) on Real-World Evidence in Healthcare Decision Making known as ISPOR-ISPE. The ISPOR-ISPE Good Practices for RWD Studies under the ISPOR/ISPE Task Force cover several topics, e.g., study registration, replicability, and stakeholder involvement, etc. (Berger et al. (2017).

The Agency for Healthcare Research and Quality (AHRQ, 2013) issued a guide to developing a protocol for observational comparative effectiveness research: "Developing a Protocol for Observational Comparative Effectiveness Research: A User's Guide," which was designed for investigators to consider such study designs to strengthen research and improve the transparency of the methods that are applied. The AHRQ is a US Federal agency tasked with improving the safety and quality of healthcare for American citizens by developing tools, increasing knowledge, and providing data required to improve the healthcare system and inform consumers, healthcare professionals and policy makers so they can make informed heathcare decisions (AHRQ, 2022).

AcademyHealth (2017) is a US organization that includes members of diverse experience, including health services researchers, policymakers, health care practitioners, and stakeholders for purposes of: (1) increasing understanding of methods and data used in the field (2) enhancing professional skills of researchers and research users, and (3) expand awareness (AHRQ, 2022). AcademyHealth's complex interventions guide examines various recommndations for study designs, which represent a mix of experimental, quasi-experimental and observational designs, e.g., randomized controlled trial, cluster randomized stepped wedge design, interrupted time series design, controlled before and after design, regression discontinuity design, and natural experiment.

A lack of ethical standards in RWE generation and use can be detrimental, further compounded by the varied RWE and RWD study types that warrant a wide variety of ethical deliberations (see: Katkade et al., 2018; Zou et al., 2020). Standards for observational studies and pragmatic clinical trials, including biomarker diagnoses / validations, genetic testing, and the thoughts and wishes of health care providers (HCPs)/patients/patients' families, are important to consider during informed consent (IC) process, particularly if a patient may have provided consent for one particular use of their data at time of consent. A standard IC process for retrospective use of RWD may still be evolving in the digital era for prospective data collection, observational, non-interventional or low-interventional RWE studies. This gray area has been the source of questions around whether such data can be used, particularly if the patient provided consent for a different study or purpose in the past. It is crucial that the IC process rely on good clinical practice (FDA, 2020).

Although there are presently no industry-wide benchmarks for ethical standards in RWE, there do exist powerful platforms built that have prompted the need to ensure human subjects' rights (and now, their data) are protected when it comes to scientific research. All such platforms are built upon strong historical foundations designed to protect the rights of human subjects involved in research, such as the Declaration of Helsinki.

3.3 Ethics Committee and Institutional Review Board

3.3.1 Historical Events Driving Ethical Research

The need to require and implement measures that ensure the safety of patients involved in clinical research has become more apparent through experience garnered over the years. This section will review historical events that underscore the significance of governance bodies, such as Ethics Committees (ECs) and Institutional Review Boards (IRBs), which exist globally and continue to evolve to ensure patients' rights are protected throughout the course of any research involving human subjects. A review of notable cases that serve as the basis for ethical conduct of research in human subjects today, are provided in the following pages.

Case Study 1: The Nuremberg Trials/the Doctors' Trial

Description: The Nuremberg Trials refers to a series of 12 military hearings held after World War II, where prominent members of political, military, judicial and economic leadership of Nazi Germany were prosecuted for war crimes related to the Holocaust (Hanauske-Abel 1996). The Doctors' trial was the first of the Nuremberg trials; this trial involved a total of twenty-three defendants, twenty of which were medical doctors, who were accused of being involved in Nazi-led human experimentation and mass murder. Nazi human experimentation was described as carrying out medical procedures that demonstrated no consideration for the health, safety, or physical and emotional suffering of the participants/victims in the experiment.

Outcome: Defendants received sentences ranging from acquittal to imprisonment or a death sentence.

Influence: The medical experiments conducted by Nazi doctors and prosecuted accordingly during the Nuremberg trials, led to the creation of the Nuremberg Code (a set of research ethics principles for human experimentation) in an effort to inform the ethical control of future trials involving human subjects. It is considered one of the most important documents in the history of ethics in the context of medical research involving humans (Shuster 1997).

Permissible Medical Experiments

The great weight of the evidence before us to effect that certain types of medical experiments on human beings, when kept within reasonably well-defined bounds, conform to the ethics of the medical profession generally. The protagonists of the practice of human experimentation justify their views on the basis that such experiments yield results for the good of society that are unprocurable by other methods or means of study. All agree, however, that certain basic principles must be observed in order to satisfy moral, ethical and legal concepts:

1. The voluntary consent of the human subject is absolutely essential. This means that the person involved should have legal capacity to give consent; should be so situated as to be able to exercise free power of choice, without the intervention of any element of force, fraud, deceit, duress, overreaching, or other ulterior form of constraint or coercion; and should have sufficient knowledge and comprehension of the elements of the subject matter involved as to enable him to make an understanding and enlightened decision. This latter element requires that before the acceptance of an affirmative decision by the experimental subject there should be made known to him the nature, duration, and purpose of the experiment; the method and means by which it is to be conducted; all inconveniences and hazards reasonably to be expected; and the effects upon his health or person which may possibly come from his participation in the experiment.

   The duty and responsibility for ascertaining the quality of the consent rests upon each individual who initiates, directs, or engages in the experiment. It is a personal duty and responsibility which may not be delegated to another with impunity.
2. The experiment should be such as to yield fruitful results for the good of society, unprocurable by other methods or means of study, and not random and unnecessary in nature.
3. The experiment should be so designed and based on the results of animal experimentation and a knowledge of the natural history of the disease or other problem under study that the anticipated results justify the performance of the experiment.
4. The experiment should be so conducted as to avoid all unnecessary physical and mental suffering and injury.
5. No experiment should be conducted where there is an a priori reason to believe that death or disabling injury will occur; except, perhaps, in those experiments where the experimental physicians also serve as subjects.
6. The degree of risk to be taken should never exceed that determined by the humanitarian importance of the problem to be solved by the experiment.
7. Proper preparations should be made and adequate facilities provided to protect the experimental subject against even remote possibilities of injury, disability or death.
8. The experiment should be conducted only by scientifically qualified persons. The highest degree of skill and care should be required through all stages of the experiment of those who conduct or engage in the experiment.
9. During the course of the experiment the human subject should be at liberty to bring the experiment to an end if he has reached the physical or mental state where continuation of the experiment seems to him to be impossible.
10. During the course of the experiment the scientist in charge must be prepared to terminate the experiment at any stage, if he has probable cause to believe, in the exercise of the good faith, superior skill and careful judgment required of him, that a continuation of the experiment is likely to result in injury, disability, or death to the experimental subject.

FIGURE 3.2
The Nuremberg Code (source: www.cirp.org/library/ethics/nuremberg/).

Decades later, the events of Nuremberg have bestowed upon modern medicine a foundation by which institutions can operate for the purpose of upholding basic human rights in clinical research. The Nuremberg Doctors' trial serves as a stark reminder to consistently apply and enforce the human rights provisions outlined in the Nuremberg Code (Figure 3.2), which ensures rights of subjects in medical research are being recognized and honored.

Case Study 2: The Tuskegee study and the Belmont report (Belmont Report, Tuskegee Study)

Description: In Alabama, US, the US Public Health Service, in partnership with the Tuskegee Institute, initiated a study in 1932 to record the natural history and progression of syphilis. The study involved N=600 African-American men, 399 of whom had syphilis. The study subjects were recruited without appropriate IC, i.e., they were not informed by researchers of the real purpose of the study. Subjects were under the impression they were being treated for "bad blood", which was a blanket term used to describe several potential ailments, including diseases ranging from syphilis to simply fatigue. Despite penicillin having been coined as a primary or first-line treatment for syphilis in the late 1940s, study subjects were not offered this or even informed about its availability, allowing their disease to progress. There was no indication that study subjects were even given a choice to quit the study.

Outcome: In July 1972, an Associated Press report about the Tuskegee Study triggered public outrage, leading to appointment of an Advisory Panel (consisting of representatives from medicine, law, religion, education, health administration, public affairs and labor) to evaluate the study. The conclusion reached by the advisory panel was that the Tuskegee study was "ethically unjustified" and that, compared to the risks imposed on subjects as a result of study conduct, the knowledge gained from the research was scant in comparison. In October 1972, the advisory panel recommended the study be stopped immediately; in November 1972, a representative from the US Health and Scientific Affairs declared the end of the Tuskegee Study.

Influence: Public outrage over the Tuskegee Study resulted in passage of the National Research Act of 1974 (Code of Federal Regulations) and the implementation of a Health and Human Services Policy for Protection of Human Research Subjects (Federal Policy for the Protection of Human Subjects). Upon enactment of these, any research in the US involving human subjects must now be reviewed and approved by an Institutional Review Board (IRB). All research requires that subjects voluntarily provide their IC to participate in the research study. IC refers to written consent from a potential research subject prior to being assigned to a treatment group; this consent confirms that the participant is fully informed and able to comprehend all aspects of the research intended to occur, including the study objectives, treatment options, risks/benefits, data collected, methods for treatment assignment, etc.

The Tuskegee Study motivated the creation of the National Commission for the Protection of Human Subjects of Biomedical and Behavioral Research; this Commission was tasked with identifying the very basic ethical principles that researchers should be held to in the context of research that involves human subjects. In 1978, the Commission identified and published what they identified to be three fundamental ethical principles to consider for all research involving human subjects: 1) Respect for Persons 2) Beneficence 3) Justice (Belmont Report, HHS.gov, 2022).

3.3.2 Modern Governance for Ethical Research

As defined by the World Health Organization (2009), a research EC is a "group of individuals who undertake the ethical review of research protocols involving humans, applying agreed ethical principles" (Das and Sil 2017, Research ethics committees: basic concepts for capacity-building). The ultimate goal of an EC is to promote the highest ethical standards in health-related research; this consists of protecting both the human rights of potential human research subjects as well as considering the impact of such research on a community. ECs can exist and operate within specific research institutions or on a regional or national basis.

The responsibilities of ECs consist of reviewing proposed research studies prior to initiation, that involve human subjects to ensure they conform to both international and local ethical guidelines. Each EC review typically consists of study protocols and patient-related documents e.g., materials used to obtain IC, confidentiality protections, etc. ECs have the authority to not only approve research, but they can also reject or stop studies based on the outcome of their review. ECs also review certain changes that occur during the conduct of a trial as well as perform standard surveillance or follow-up after the end of research, as applicable.

ECs are typically composed of individuals that have medical and scientific expertise, which will allow for the appropriate identification and evaluation of the risks and benefits associated with the research at hand as well as the scientific validity of the study's proposed design. ECs are supplemented with representatives that possess social, cultural or legal education or experience that could inform the evaluation. EC members receive training in applicable ethical and legal standards that govern human research (internationally and locally) as well as those processes specific to that EC.

Similar to ECs, an IRB possesses the responsibility, diverse membership and oversight (before and throughout conduct of a study) when it comes to research involving human subjects. The terms IRB and EC are often used interchangeably; IRB is a term more commonly used in the US whereas ECs are more commonly referred to in the EU or ex-US. These IRB bodies may be referred to differently in certain parts of the world depending on local law and jurisdiction. Under US FDA's regulations, an IRB "is an appropriately constituted group that has been formally designated to review and monitor biomedical research involving human subjects" (Information sheet, Guidance for Institutional Review Boards and Clinical Investigators, January 1998). IRBs are responsible for ensuring that appropriate measures are taken to protect the rights and welfare of all human subjects participating in research. IRBs have the authority to request modifications to planned research for purposes of approval or, on the contrary, to disapprove research. IRBs make their decisions based on review of relevant clinical trial materials, including the protocol, IC documents and investigator brochures. Per 21 CFR Part 56, each IRB in the US that reviews FDA-regulated studies must register with FDA prior to approving research studies (21 CFR 56.106). According to the US Department of Health and Human Services (DHHS) Office for Human Research Protections (OHRP), there are some exemptions to IRB oversight; however, such exemptions are typically decided case by case and by an IRB representative rather than an investigator involved directly in specific research (Code of Federal Regulations). Exemptions include research performed in conventional educational settings, research involving analysis of existing data or materials that are in the public domain or where the data exist in a manner where the subject providing the data cannot be identified and research designed to assess effectiveness of a public benefit/service program (Code of Federal Regulations).

ECs, IRBs, or similar bodies are required widely around the world in accordance with local laws and jurisdictions (Grady, 2015). In the US, institutions that conduct research of their own can typically have their own IRBs; however, regulations in the US permit institutions to arrange for an external IRB (independent or institutional) for purposes of reviewing and approving the research. Independent review of clinical research by an IRB is required for any US study involving research or testing of drugs, biologics and devices, which fall within the jurisdiction of the US FDA. These include studies funded by the DHHS and other US federal agencies (Grady 2015).

In addition to an active oversight of clinical research to ensure the research is carried out in an ethical fashion, laws have been enacted to enforce the rights of humans with respect to privacy and human data protection. Two well-known related laws include the HIPAA in the US, and the GDPR in the EU (refer Section 3.1 above). As with any other research study, it is expected that ethical principles are applied to studies performed in the realm of RWE, particularly for prospective primary data-collection studies. In other words, when it comes to utilization of an individual's data, personal rights to those data must be protected, while the subject must be fully informed and provide consent to any use of their personal data for research purposes (unless the data are truly de-identified).

3.4 Best Practices

3.4.1 Understand Data and Craft Analysis Plan

Clarity around the purpose, scope, features, and limitations of datasets for specific context of use is important and should be considered a best practice for protecting privacy and ethical research in the RWE space. The 21st Century Cures Act that defined RWE, for example, expresses the need for clarity about how data can be used and where data can be made available (21st Century Cures Act, FDA 2020). The legislation language in the US, for example, states that the data must not contain individually identifiable health information and should be research-identifiable files.

It can be useful to communicate with patients regarding their symptoms or the impact of a disease or condition on the concept of interest as well as which digital tools are intended to be used for patient-reported outcome measurements (e.g. electronic surveys). It is important to thoroughly consider the purposes of the observational studies or pragmatic trials before embarking on development of research questions or testing a priori hypotheses, specifically to ensure that any patient or subject is appropriately informed about how their data will be used and for what purpose(s). The Agency for Healthcare Research and Quality has developed a user's guide for developing a protocol for observational studies (Developing a Protocol for Observational Comparative Effectiveness Research, AHRQ, 2013).

3.4.2 Share Data via Distributed Research Network

The National Institutes of Health's (NIH) Collaboratory Distributed Research Network (DRN) enables investigators to collaborate with each other in the use of electronic health data, while also safeguarding protected health information and proprietary data (NIH Collaboratory Distributed Research Network). It supports both single- and multisite research programs. The DRN fully leverages the FDA Sentinel System's data, methods, tools, and querying infrastructure. It can also directly contact providers and health plan members to collect new information or in support of randomized clinical trials (FDA's Sentinel Initiative 2019).

The Network's querying capabilities reduce the need to share confidential or proprietary data by enabling authorized researchers to send queries to collaborators holding data (i.e., data partners).

In some cases, queries can take the form of computer programs that a data partner can execute on a pre-existing dataset. The data partner can return the query result, typically aggregated (count) data, rather than the data itself. This form of remote querying reduces legal, regulatory, privacy, proprietary, and technical barriers associated with data sharing for research. The network seeks to build strong and trusted collaborations to support the research that will lead to improved health for millions of people around the world (e.g., see BBCIC, 2022).

3.4.3 Leverage Available Tools and RWE Guidance Documents

To date, health authorities around the world are realizing the potential and application of RWE and are responding to this enthusiasm by issuing guidance to industry, which includes important considerations for ensuring ethical use of such information for the advancement of science. In the US, the FDA has developed a framework for an RWE program (Real-World Evidence, US FDA 2021, FDA in brief 2019, California Consumer Privacy Act). There are several guidance documents, including the "Use of Electronic Health Records in Clinical Investigations," "Use of Real-World Evidence to Support Regulatory Decision-Making for Medical Devices," "Submitting Documents Utilizing Real-World Data and Real-World Evidence to FDA for Drugs and Biologics, Developing Real-World Data and Evidence to Support Regulatory Decision-Making." FDA has also announced a new Sentinel system contract, affirming its commitment to harnessing RWD to improve the safety and effectiveness of drugs. For data privacy protection, there is also the "California Consumer Privacy Act" (CCPA).

In other parts of the world, such as the EU, the EMA has issued its "Regulatory Perspective on Real-world Evidence (RWE) in Scientific Advice (Mosely 2018)." The EMA (2020) created a joint big data task force to describe the big data landscape from a regulatory viewpoint and to help identify steps for those in the European healthcare network to leverage big data for purposes of facilitating innovation and public health in the EU. The EMA is preparing a big data Q&A guidance specifically to help medicine developers, data providers and research bodies comply with EU data protection rules and to help patients understand their rights and existing safeguards to protect their persona information (Regulatory Affairs Professionals Society, 2020). In China, the CDE, MNPA has issued "Key Considerations in Using Real-World Evidence to Support Drug Development." Japan's PMDA discussed "Recent Trend on Utilization of Real-world Data Challenges in Japan."

Remarks

RWD includes many types of non-RCT data sources, which pose challenges and opportunities associated with regulatory use and ethical considerations. Such challenges co-exist, especially in the regulatory landscapes associated with health-related outcome studies and analyses. Findings measured by those outcomes may be used to support claims in approved medical product labeling when the claims are derived from adequate and well-controlled investigations in which PROs measure specific concepts accurately and as intended. Such instruments can be developed and assessed in accordance with regulatory guidance documents from the FDA and EMA.

To bring value to patients, healthcare providers, and payers, industry must think strategically, work scientifically and communicate effectively. It is clear that regulatory entities actively protect patient data privacy and PHI; however, a unified approach to ethical and bioethical standards within or across sectors for utilization of RWD and RWE must be further examined, developed and elevated in order to ensure effective application.

Disclaimer

Corinne S. Pillai, Kelly H. Zou, and Ewa Filipowska are employees of Viatris, merged between Upjohn, a Division of Pfizer, and Mylan. Eleanor E. Panico is former employee of Upjohn, a Division of Pfizer, and Viatris. The views expressed are the authors' own and do not necessarily represent those of their employer or employers. The authors appreciate the editorial support from Arghya Bhattacharya and Aswin Kumar A of Viatris.

References

AcademyHealth. Evaluating Complex Health Interventions: A Guide to Rigorous Research Designs. 2017. www.academyhealth.org/evaluationguide (Accessed on March 30, 2022).

AcademyHealth. Evaluating Complex Health Interventions: A Guide to Rigorous Research Designs. 2017. www.academyhealth.org/evaluationguide (Accessed on March 30, 2022).

Agency for Healthcare Research and Quality. Developing a Protocol for Observational Comparative Effectiveness Research: A User's Guide. 2013. www.effectivehealthcare.ahrq.gov/index.cfm/search-for-guides-reviews-and-reports/?pageaction=displayproduct&productid=1166&pcem=ra (Accessed on March 30, 2022).

Agency for Healthcare Research and Quality. Developing a Protocol for Observational Comparative Effectiveness Research: A User's Guide. Eds. Velentgas P, Dreyer NA, Nourjah P, Smith SR, Torchia MM. 2013. https://effectivehealthcare.ahrq.gov/sites/default/files/related_files/user-guide-observational-cer-130113.pdf (Accessed on March 30, 2022).

Agency for Healthcare Research and Quality. AHRQ. Agency for Healthcare Research and Quality: A Profile. 2022. www.ahrq.gov/cpi/about/profile/index.html (Accessed on March 30, 2022).

Agency for Healthcare Research and Quality. Developing a Protocol for Observational Comparative Effectiveness Research: A User's Guide. Eds. Velentgas P, Dreyer NA, Nourjah P, Smith SR, Torchia MM. 2013. https://effectivehealthcare.ahrq.gov/sites/default/files/related_files/user-guide-observational-cer-130113.pdf (Accessed on March 30, 2022).

Alemayehu D, Berger M. Big Data: transforming drug development and health policy decision making. Health Serv Outcomes Res Method. 2016. DOI 10.1007/s10742-016-0144-x.

Althof SE, Cappelleri JC, Shpilsky A, Stecher V, Diuguid C, Sweeney M, and S Duttagupta. Treatment responsiveness of the Self-Esteem And Relationship (SEAR) questionnaire in erectile dysfunction. Urology. 2003; 61:888–893.

Annemans L, Aristides M, Kubin M. Real-Life Data: A Growing Need, ISPOR Connections 2007.

Baker CL, Zou KH, Su J. Long-acting bronchodilator use after hospitalization for COPD: an observational study of health insurance claims data. Int J Chron Obstruct Pulmon Dis. 2014 May 3;9:431–439.

BBCIC. Org. BBCIC Governance. 2022. www.bbcic.org/about/bbcic-governance (Accessed on March 30, 2022).

Berger ML, Doban V. Big data, advanced analytics and the future of comparative effectiveness research. J Comp Eff Res. 2014 Mar;3(2):167–176.

Berger ML, Sox H, Willke RJ, Brixner DL, Eichler HG, Goettsch W, Madigan D, Makady A, Schneeweiss S, Tarricone R, Wang SV, Watkins J, Daniel Mullins C. Good practices for real-world data studies of treatment and/or comparative effectiveness: Recommendations from the joint ISPOR-ISPE Special Task Force on real-world evidence in health care decision making. Pharmacoepidemiol Drug Saf. 2017;26(9):1033–1039.

Berger ML, Sox H, Willke RJ, Brixner DL, Eichler HG, Goettsch W, Madigan D, Makady A, Schneeweiss S, Tarricone R, Wang SV, Watkins J, Daniel Mullins C. Good practices for real-world data studies of treatment and/or comparative effectiveness: Recommendations from the joint ISPOR-ISPE Special Task Force on real-world evidence in health care decision making. Pharmacoepidemiol Drug Saf. 2017;26(9):1033–1039.

Biotechnology Innovation Organization. Incorporating real-world evidence within the label of an FDA-approved drug: perspectives from bio membership. 2019. www.bio.org/sites/default/files/legacy/bioorg/docs/BIO%20White%20paper%20%20-%20Incorporating%20RWE%20Within%20the%20Label_FINAL%202019.pdf (Accessed on March 30, 2022).

Boston University School of Public Health. Institutional Review Boards and the Belmont Principles. 2022. https://sphweb.bumc.bu.edu/otlt/mph-modules/ep/ep713_researchethics/ep713_researchethics3.html (Accessed on March 30, 2022).

Burns PB, Rohrich RJ, Chung KC. The levels of evidence and their role in evidence-based medicine. Plast Reconstr Surg 2011;128:305–310.

Cappelleri JC, Zou KH, Bushmakin AG, Alvir JMJ, Alemayehu D and T Symonds. Patient-reported outcomes: Measurement, implementation and interpretation. 2013. Boca Raton, FL: Chapman & Hall/CRC Press (Taylor & Francis).

Cattell J, Groves P, Hughes B, Savas S. How can pharmacos take advantage of the real-world data opportunity in healthcare. McKinsey & Company. IT Insight. 2011.

Centers for Disease Control and Prevention. Health Insurance Portability and Accountability Act of 1996 (HIPAA). 2022a. www.cdc.gov/phlp/publications/topic/hipaa.html. (Accessed on March 30, 2022).

Centers for Disease Control and Prevention. Tuskegee Study-timeline, Centres for disease control and prevention. 2022b. www.cdc.gov/tuskegee/timeline.htm (Accessed on March 30, 2022).

Cheung C, Bietz MJ, Patrick K and Bloss CS. Privacy attitudes among early adopters of emerging health technologies. PloS one, 2016; 11(11), p.e0166389.

Cohen A, Goto S, Schreiber K, Torp-Pedersen C. Why do we need observational studies of everyday patients in the real-life setting? European Heart Journal Supplements 2015;17:D2-D8.

Das NK and Sil A, 2017. Evolution of ethics in clinical research and ethics committee. Indian Journal of Dermatology, 62(4), p.373.

de Vet HCW, Terwee CB, Mokkink LB and DL Knol. Measurement in Medicine: A practical guide. New York, NY: Cambridge University Press. 2011.

European Commission. European Health Data Space. 2022a. https://ec.europa.eu/health/ehealth-digital-health-and-care/european-health-data-space_en (Accessed on May 3. 2022).

European Commission. Questions and Answers - EU Health: European Health Data Space (EHDS). 2022b. https://ec.europa.eu/commission/presscorner/detail/en/QANDA_22_2712 (Accessed on May 3, 2022).

European Medicines Agency. Big Data. 2022. https://www.ema.europa.eu/en/about-us/how-we-work/big-data (Accessed on March 30, 2022).

Food & Drug Administration. Center for Devices and Radiological Health (CDRH). December 2009. www.fda.gov/media/77832/download (Accessed on March 30, 2022).

Food & Drug Administration. 21st Century Cures Act. 2020a. www.fda.gov/regulatory-information/selected-amendments-fdc-act/21st-century-cures-act (Accessed on March 30, 2022).

Food & Drug Administration. E6(R2) Good Clinical Practice: Integrated Addendum to ICH E6(R1). 2020b. www.fda.gov/files/drugs/published/E6%28R2%29-Good-Clinical-Practice--Integrated-Addendum-to-ICH-E6%28R1%29.pdf (Accessed on March 30, 2022).

Food & Drug Administration. FDA Issues Draft Guidances on Real-World Evidence, Prepares to Publish More in Future. 2022. www.fda.gov/drugs/news-events-human-drugs/fda-issues-draft-guidances-real-world-evidence-prepares-publish-more-future#:~:text=for%20Human%20Drugs-,FDA%20Issues%20Draft%20Guidances%20on%20Real%2DWorld%20Evidence%2C%20Prepares,to%20Publish%20More%20in%20Future&text=Collection%20and%20analysis%20of%20real,of%20RWD's%20strengths%20and%20limitations (Accessed on March 30, 2020).

European Data Protection Supervisor, The History of the General Data Protection Regulation. 2022. https://edps.europa.eu/data-protection/data-protection/legislation/history-general-data-protection-regulation_en (Accessed on March 30, 2022).

EUR-Lex. Protection of personal data (from 2018). 2022. https://eur-lex.europa.eu/legal-content/EN/LSU/?uri=CELEX:32016R0679 (Accessed on March 30, 2022).

European Medicines Agency. Opinions and letters of support on the qualification of novel methodologies for medicine development. 2022, www.ema.europa.eu/ema/index.jsp?curl=pages/regulation/document_listing/document_listing_000319.jsp (Accessed on March 30, 2022).

European Medicines Agency. European Medicines Agencies Network Strategy to 2025: Protecting Public Health at a Time of Rapid Change. 2020. www.ema.europa.eu/en/documents/report/european-union-medicines-agencies-network-strategy-2025-protecting-public-health-time-rapid-change_en.pdf (Accessed on March 30, 2022).

European Medicines Agency. European Medicines Agencies Network Strategy to 2025: Protecting Public Health at a Time of Rapid Change (Draft). July 2020. www.ema.europa.eu/en/documents/other/european-medicines-agencies-network-strategy-2025-protecting-public-health-time-rapid-change_en.pdf (Accessed on March 30, 2022).

European Medicine Agency. European Medicines Agencies Network Strategy to 2025: Protecting Public Health at a Time of Rapid Change (Draft). 2020. www.ema.europa.eu/en/documents/other/european-medicines-agencies-network-strategy-2025-protecting-public-health-time-rapid-change_en.pdf (Accessed on March 30, 2022).

European Medicines Agency (EMA), Committee for Medicinal Products for Human Use. 2005. Reflection paper on the regulatory guidance for us of health-related quality of life (HRQOL) measures in the evaluation of medicinal products. European Medicines Agency.

European Union. General Data Protection Regulation (GDPR). 2020. https://gdpr.eu/tag/gdpr (Accessed on March 30, 2022).

European Medicines Agency. Qualification of novel methodologies for drug development: guidance to applicants. 2014. www.ema.europa.eu/en/documents/regulatory-procedural-guideline/qualification-novel-methodologies-drug-development-guidance-applicants_en.pdf (Accessed on March 30, 2022).

European Medicines Agency. Big Data. 2022. www.ema.europa.eu/en/about-us/how-we-work/big-data#main-content (Accessed on March 30, 2022).

European Parliament. Fact Sheets on the European Union: Personal data protection. 2022.www.europarl.europa.eu/factsheets/en/sheet/157/personal-data-protection (Accessed on March 30, 2022).

Fennema-Notestine C, Ozyurt IB, Clark CP, Morris S, Bischoff-Grethe A, Bondi MW, Jernigan TL, Fischl B, Segonne F, Shattuck DW, Leahy RM, Rex DE, Toga AW, Zou KH, Brown GG. Quantitative evaluation of automated skull-stripping methods applied to contemporary and legacy images: effects of diagnosis, bias correction, and slice location. Hum Brain Mapp. 2006;27(2):99–113.

Food & Drug Administration. FDA in Brief: FDA announces a new Sentinel System contract, affirming its commitment to harnessing Real-World Data to improve the safety and effectiveness of drugs, US FDA 2019. www.fda.gov/news-events/fda-brief/fda-brief-fda-announces-new-sentinel-system-contract-affirming-its-commitment-harnessing-real-world?utm_campaign=092719_FIB_FDA%20announces%20a%20new%20Sentinel%20System%20contract&utm_medium=email&utm_source=Eloqua (Accessed on March 30, 2022).

Food & Drug Administration. FDA's Sentinel Initiative, 2019. www.fda.gov/safety/fdas-sentinel-initiative (Accessed on March 30, 2022).

Food & Drug Administration. Patient-Reported Outcome Measures: Use in Medical Product Development to Support Labeling Claims. 2009. www.fda.gov/regulatory-information/search-fda-guidance-documents/patient-reported-outcome-measures-use-medical-product-development-support-labeling-claims (Accessed on March 30, 2022).

Food & Drug Administration. Qualification Process for Drug Development Tools Guidance for Industry and FDA Staff. www.fda.gov/regulatory-information/search-fda-guidance-documents/qualification-process-drug-development-tools-guidance-industry-and-fda-staff (Accessed on March 30, 2022).

Food & Drug Administration. Framework for FDA's Real-World Evidence Program. December 2018b. www.fda.gov/media/120060/download (Accessed on March 30, 2022).

Food & Drug Administration. Use of Electronic Health Record Data in Clinical Investigations Guidance for Industry. 2018. www.fda.gov/regulatory-information/search-fda-guidance-documents/use-electronic-health-record-data-clinical-investigations-guidance-industry (Accessed on March 30, 2022).

Food & Drug Administration. Use of Real-World Evidence to Support Regulatory Decision-Making for Medical Devices. 2017. www.fda.gov/regulatory-information/search-fda-guidance-documents/use-real-world-evidence-support-regulatory-decision-making-medical-devices (Accessed on March 30, 2022).

Food & Drug Administration. Submitting Documents Using Real-World Data and Real-World Evidence to FDA for Drugs and Biologics: Guidance for Industry, US FDA, 2019, www.fda.gov/regulatory-information/search-fda-guidance-documents/submitting-documents-using-real-world-data-and-real-world-evidence-fda-drugs-and-biologics-guidance (Accessed on March 30, 2022).

Food & Drug Administration. FDA Issues Draft Guidances on Real-World Evidence, Prepares to Publish More in Future. 2022a. www.fda.gov/drugs/news-events-human-drugs/fda-issues-draft-guidances-real-world-evidence-prepares-publish-more-future#:~:text=for%20Human%20Drugs-,FDA%20Issues%20Draft%20Guidances%20on%20Real%2DWorld%20Evidence%2C%20Prepares,to%20Publish%20More%20in%20Future&text=Collection%20and%20analysis%20of%20real,of%20RWD's%20strengths%20and%20limitations. (Accessed on March 30, 2020).

Food & Drug Administration. Drug Development Tool (DDT) Qualification Programs. 2022b. www.fda.gov/drugs/development-approval-process-drugs/drug-development-tool-ddt-qualification-programs (Accessed on March 30, 2022).

Food & Drug Administration. Real-World Evidence. 2022c. www.fda.gov/science-research/science-and-research-special-topics/real-world-evidence (Accessed on March 30, 2022).

Garrison LP, Jr., Neumann PJ, Erickson P, Marshall D, Mullins CD. Using real-world data for coverage and payment decisions: the ISPOR Real-World Data Task Force report. Value Health 2007;10:326–335.

Goldman HB, Anger JT, Esinduy CB, Zou KH, Russell D, Luo X, Ntanios F, Carlsson MO, Clemens JQ. Real-World Patterns of Care for the Overactive Bladder Syndrome in the United States. Urology. 2016 Jan;87:64-9.

Grady, C. Institutional review boards: Purpose and challenges. Chest, 148(5), 2015;1148–1155.

Groves P, Kayyali B, Knott D, Van Kuiken S. The 'big data' revolution in healthcare. McKinsey& Company, Center for US Health System Reform Business Technology Office 2013.

Government of Canada. Personal Information Protection and Electronic Documents Act: S.C. 2000, c.5. 2020. https://laws-lois.justice.gc.ca/ENG/ACTS/P-8.6/page-1.html (Accessed on March 30, 2022).

Hanauske-Abel HM Not a slippery slope or sudden subversion: German medicine and National Socialism in 1933. BMJ, 313(7070), 1996;1453–1463.

HHS.gov. Federal Policy for the Protection of Human Subjects ('Common Rule'). 2022a. www.hhs.gov/ohrp/regulations-and-policy/regulations/common-rule/index.html (Accessed on March 30, 2022).

HHS.gov. Office for Human Research Protections. The Belmont Report: Ethical Principles and Guidelines fror the Protection of Human Subjects of Rseearch. 2022b. www.hhs.gov/ohrp/regulations-and-policy/belmont-report/index.html (Accessed on March 30, 2022).

HHS.gov. Summary of the HIPAA privacy rules. 2022c. www.hhs.gov/hipaa/for-professionals/privacy/laws-regulations/index.html (Accessed on March 30, 2022).

Holtorf AP, Watkins JB, Mullins CD, Brixner D. Incorporating observational data into the formulary decision-making process--summary of a roundtable discussion. J Manag Care Pharm 2008;14:302–308.

Food & Drug Administration. Institutional Review Boards Frequently Asked Questions, Guidance for Institutional Review Boards and Clinical Investigators, January 1998. www.fda.gov/regulatory-information/search-fda-guidance-documents/institutional-review-boards-frequently-asked-questions, (Accessed on March 30, 2022).

Food & Drug Administration. FDA Issues Draft Guidances on Real-World Evidence, Prepares to Publish More in Future. 2022 www.fda.gov/drugs/news-events-human-drugs/fda-issues-draft-guidances-real-world-evidence-prepares-publish-more-future#:~:text=for%20Human%20Drugs-,FDA%20Issues%20Draft%20Guidances%20on%20Real%2DWorld%20Evidence%2C%20Prepares,to%20Publish%20More%20in%20Future&text=Collection%20and%20analysis%20of%20real,of%20RWD's%20strengths%20and%20limitations. (Accessed on March 30, 2020).

Katkade VB, Sanders KN, Zou KH. Real world data: an opportunity to supplement existing evidence for the use of long-established medicines in health care decision making. J Multidiscip Healthc. 2018 2;11:295–304.

KPMG. Overview of China's Cybersecurity Law. February 2017. https://assets.kpmg/content/dam/kpmg/cn/pdf/en/2017/02/overview-of-cybersecurity-law.pdf (Accessed on March 30, 2022).

Makady A, van Veelen A, Jonsson P, Moseley O, D'Andon A, de Boer A, Hillege H, Klungel O and Goettsch W Using real-world data in health technology assessment (HTA) practice: a comparative study of five HTA agencies. Pharmacoeconomics, 2018: 36(3);359–368.

Miani C, Robin E, Veronika Horvath V et al. Health and Healthcare: Assessing the Real-World Data Policy Landscape in Europe 2014.

Moseley J. Regulatory Perspective on Real World Evidence (RWE) in scientific advice, EMA Human Scientific Committees' Working Parties with Patients' and Consumers' Organisations (PCWP) and Healthcare Professionals' Organisations (HCPWP) 2018. www.ema.europa.eu/en/documents/presentation/presentation-regulatory-perspective-real-world-evidence-rwe-scientific-advice-emas-pcwp-hcpwp-joint_en.pdf (Accessed on March 30, 2022).

National Archives. Code of Federal Regulations Title 21, www.ecfr.gov/ (Accessed on March 30, 2022). 23.

National Archives. Code of Federal Regulations, PART 46 – PROTECTION OF HUMAN SUBJECTS 2022. www.ecfr.gov/current/title-45/subtitle-A/subchapter-A/part-46 (Accessed on March 30, 2022).

Network for Excellence in Health Innovation. Real-World Evidence: A New Era for Health Care Innovation 2015. www.nehi-us.org/publications/66-real-world-evidence-a-new-era-for-health-care-innovation/view#:~:text=A%20new%20era%20of%20health,multiple%20sources%20of%20diverse%20data. (Accessed on March 30, 2022).

New America. Translation: Cybersecurity Law of the People's Republic of China (Effective June 1, 2017). 2018. www.newamerica.org/cybersecurity-

NIH Pragmatic Trials Collaboratory: Rethinking Clinical Trials. NIH Collaboratory Distributed Research Network (DRN): Millions of people. Strong collaborations. Privacy first. 2022. https://rethinkingclinicaltrials.org/nih-collaboratory-drn (Accessed on March 30, 2022).

Office of the Privacy Commissioner of Canada. The Personal Information Protection and Electronic Documents Act (PIPEDA). 2022. www.priv.gc.ca/en/privacy-topics/privacy-laws-in-canada/the-personal-information-protection-and-electronic-documents-act-pipeda/pipeda_brief/ (Accessed on March 30, 2022).

Patrick DL, Burke LB, Gwaltney CH, Kline Leidy N, Martin ML, Molsen E, and L Ring. 2011b. Content Validity – Establishing and reporting the evidence in newly developed patient reported outcomes (PRO) instruments for medical product evaluation: ISPOR PRO good research practices task force report: Part 2 – Assessing respondent understanding. Value Health 14:978–988.

Private Analytics, an IQVIA Company. GDPR and Anonymization, 2020. https://privacy-analytics.com/resources/white-papers/gdpr-and-anonymization/ (Accessed on March 30, 2022).

Publications Office of the European Union. Regulation (EU) 2016/679 of the European Parliament and of the Council of 27 April 2016 on the protection of natural persons with regard to the processing of personal data and on the free movement of such data, and repealing Directive 95/46/EC (General Data Protection Regulation) (Text with EEA relevance) (OJ L 119 04.05.2016, p. 1, CELEX. 2016. https://eur-lex.europa.eu/legal-content/EN/TXT/?uri=CELEX:32016R0679 (Accessed on March 30, 2022).

Regulatory Affairs Professionals Society. EMA preparing big data Q&A guidance. 2020. www.raps.org/news-and-articles/news-articles/2020/5/ema-preparing-big-data-qa-guidance (Accessed on March 30, 2022.

Shuster E.. Fifty years later: the significance of the Nuremberg Code. New England Journal of Medicine, 1997; 337(20):1436–1440.

Streiner DL, Norman GR and J Cairney. 2015. Health measurement scales: A practical guide to their development and use. Fifth edition. New York, NY: Oxford University Press.

The State Council, The People's Republic of China. China to boost big data application in health and medical sectors. 2016. http://english.www.gov.cn/policies/latest_releases/2016/06/24/content_281475379018156.htm (Accessed on March 30, 2022).

UnitedHealth Group. Harvard Study Finds Value-Based Care Has a Third Critical Dimension, 2019. www.unitedhealthgroup.com/newsroom/posts/2019-10-02-havard-study-vbc.html (Accessed on March 30, 2022).

initiative/digichina/blog/translation-cybersecurity-law-peoples-republic-china (Accessed on March 30, 2022).

Stanford University. DigiChina. Translation: Data Security Law of the People's Republic of China (Effective Sept. 1, 2021). 2021. https://digichina.stanford.edu/work/translation-data-security-law-of-the-peoples-republic-of-china (Accessed on March 30, 2022).

United Nations Development Group. Data Privacy, Ethics and Protection: Guidance Note on Big Data for Achievement of the 2030 Agenda. 2020. https://unsdg.un.org/sites/default/files/UNDG_BigData_final_web.pdf. (Accessed on March 30, 2022).

Vandenbroucke JP, von Elm E, Altman DG, Gøtzsche PC, Mulrow CD, Pocock SJ, Poole C, Schlesselman JJ, Egger M. STROBE initiative. Strengthening the Reporting of Observational Studies in Epidemiology (STROBE): explanation and elaboration. Ann Intern Med. 2007 Oct 16;147(8):W163–94.

Wellcome Trust. The One-Way Mirror: Public attitudes to commercial access to health data: report prepared for the Wellcome Trust. 2016. . https://wellcome.org/sites/default/files/public-attitudes-to-commercial-access-to-health-data-wellcome-mar16.pdf (Accessed on March 30, 2022).

GDPR.EU. What is GDPR, the EU's new data protection law? 2022. https://gdpr.eu/what-is-gdpr/?cn-reloaded=1 (Accessed on March 30, 2022).

State of California Department of Justice. California Consumer Privacy Act (CCPA), Available at: https://oag.ca.gov/privacy/ccpa (Accessed on March 30, 2022).

Willke RJ, Mullins CD. "Ten commandments" for conducting comparative effectiveness research using "real-world data". J Manag Care Pharm 2011;17:S10–5.

World Health Organization. Research ethics committees: basic concepts for capacity-building., World Health Organization 2009. www.who.int/ethics/Ethics_basic_concepts_ENG.pdf (Accessed on March 30, 2022).

World Medical Association. World Medical Association Declaration of Helsinki: ethical principles for medical research involving human subjects. JAMA. 2013 Nov 27; 310(20):2191–4.

Yamada K. Big Data Utilization for Post-Marketing Drug Safety Measures in Japan. PMDA. 2020. www.pmda.go.jp/files/000221711.pdf (Accessed on March 30, 2022).

Yamaguchi M, Inomata S, Harada S, Matsuzaki Y, Kawaguchi M, Ujibe M, Kishiba M, Fujimura Y, Kimura M, Murata K, Nakashima N, Nakayama M, Ohe K, Orii T, Sueoka E, Suzuki T, Yokoi H, Takahashi F, Uyama Y. Establishment of the MID-NET® medical information database network as a reliable and valuable database for drug safety assessments in Japan. Pharmacoepidemiol Drug Saf. 2019;28(10):1395–1404. doi: 10.1002/pds.4879.

Zikopoulos PC, Eaton C, deRoos D, Deutsch T, Lapis G. Understanding Big Data. New York: McGraw Hill; 2012.

Zou KH, Li JZ, Imperato J, Potkar CN, Sethi N, Edwards J, Ray A. Harnessing real-world data for regulatory use and applying innovative applications. J Multidiscip Healthc. 2020;13:671–679.

4

Real-World Data, Big Data, and Artificial Intelligence: Recent Development and Emerging Trends in the European Union

Kelly H. Zou
Viatris

CONTENTS

4.1 Introduction

Real-world evidence (RWE) is increasingly gaining importance in the regulatory framework of the European Union (EU). The Heads of Medicines Agencies (HMA) and European Medicines Agencies (EMA) have recently held several workshops, focusing on big data and artificial intelligence as key initiatives. The EMA has issued a number of guidance documents for leveraging real-world data (RWD) in the areas of medical evidence generation and regulatory approval. Given the constantly evolving landscape and increasing

DOI: 10.1201/9781003017523-4

uses of RWE, it is useful to summarize the policies and strategies for RWD and big data in the EU.

4.2 Network Strategy

The EMA's network strategy outlines the following six overarching priority focus areas via EU's roadmap for a pharmaceutical strategy (EMA, 2020).

- Availability and accessibility of medicines
- Data analytics, digital tools and digital transformation
- Innovation
- Antimicrobial resistance and other emerging health threats
- Supply-chain challenges
- Sustainability of the network and operational excellence

The regulator has emphasized that "the Network will always attempt to follow its broad guiding principles of trustworthiness, acting transparently, communicating clearly, ensuring the highest ethical standards, and supporting environmental sustainability through reduced use of resources, emissions, degradation and pollution related to pharmaceuticals" (EMA, 2020).

4.3 RWD, RWE, and RCTs

The European regulators have set the vision of enabling the use of RWE and establishing its value for regulatory decision-making on the development, authorization and supervision of medicines in Europe by 2025 (EMA, 2021). Besides envisioning the complementary evidence from both randomized controlled trials (RCTs) and RWE, the EMA is also interested in exploring and evaluating the potential role of RWD for new products and indication expansions (EMA, 2022b; Arlett et al., 2022; Flynn et al., 2022; Cave et al., 2019).

In EMA's perspective, specifically, the term RWD is defined as "routinely collected data relating to a patient's health status or the delivery of health care from a variety of sources other than traditional clinical trials" (Cave et al., 2019; Arlett et al., 2020). RWE is then the information derived from an analysis of RWD (Arlett et al., 2020).

Because the RCTs are considered as the gold standard along the evidence hierarchy, the EMA believes "that the binary discussion between clinical trials and RWE is unhelpful as each approach brings its own strengths and weaknesses." In other words, the EMA "embrace[s] a complementary evidence approach rather than seeing the two as being in opposition." It aims at "working on multiple fronts to establish the evidentiary value of RWE." To evaluate the value added by using RWE besides RCT, it seeks "to understand when a randomized clinical trial and when RWE is best placed to provide robust, decision-ready evidence."

Thus, the value proposition, as well as the aspects of data, methodologies and applications, are progressing and evolving (EMA, 2021), as well as the European Health Data Space (EU Commission, 2022a; EU Commission, 2022b).

4.4 Big Data

The EU's OPerational, TechnIcal, and MethodologicAL framework (OPTIMAL) framework for RWE consists of three pillars: operational, technical and methodological. Such framework consists of (1) Objective; (2) Desired criteria for acceptability of RWE; (3) Challenges with use of RWD to generate acceptable RWE; (4) Possible solutions (EU context) (Cave et al., 2019). Here, the EU views RWD in the context of big data, where

> Big data refers to large amounts of data produced very quickly by a high number of diverse sources. Data can either be created by people or generated by machines, such as sensors gathering climate information, satellite imagery, digital pictures and videos, purchase transaction records, GPS signals, and more. It covers many sectors, from healthcare to transport to energy.

EU's Big Data Task Force has initiated and implemented the following workplan (Arlett et al., 2022):

- DARWIN EU
- Data quality
- Data discoverability
- Skills
- Business processes
- Analytics capabilities
- Expert advice
- Data governance
- International collaboration
- Stakeholder engagement
- Veterinary data strategy

In terms of the value-adds of analyzing big data, the EU considers the following benefits (EMA, 2022a; EMA, 2022b):

- Transform Europe's service industries by generating a wide range of innovative information products and services
- Increase the productivity of all sectors of the economy through improved business intelligence
- Address more efficiently many of the challenges that face our societies
- Improve research and speed up innovation
- Achieve cost reductions through more personalized services
- Increase efficiency in the public sector

4.5 DARWIN EU®

Data Analysis and Real World Interrogation Network (DARWIN EU®) is a high-priority resource for big data analysis for the EU, which aligns with the EMA's Network Strategy to 2025. The EMA's a coordination center aims to "provide timely and reliable evidence on the use, safety and effectiveness of medicines for human use, including vaccines, from real world healthcare databases" across the EU (EMA, 2022b).

DARWIN EU will support regulatory decision-making by (EMA, 2022b)

- Establishing and expanding a catalogue of observational data sources for use in medicines regulation
- Providing a source of high-quality, validated real world data on the uses, safety and efficacy of medicines
- Addressing specific questions by carrying out high-quality, non-interventional studies, including developing scientific protocols, interrogating relevant data sources and interpreting and reporting study results

EMA is the principal user of DARWIN EU and will also play a central role in developing, launching and maintaining it by (EU, 2022a)

- Providing strategic direction and setting standards
- Overseeing the coordination centre and monitoring its performance
- Ensuring close links to European Commission policy initiatives, particularly the European Health Data Space (EDHS), and delivering pilots
- Reporting to EMA's Management Board, the HMA and European Commission

4.6 GDPR

EU's General Data Protection Regulation (GDPR) is the most rigorous and strict privacy and security law globally. The GDPR "imposes obligations onto organizations anywhere, so long as they target or collect data related to people in the EU."

Consequently, the GDPR levies "harsh fines against those who violate its privacy and security standards, with penalties reaching into the tens of millions of euros."

In terms of legal aspects, comprehensive details may be found on the following (GDPR.EU, 2022):

- Data protection principles
- Accountability
- Data security
- Data protection by design and by default
- When you're allowed to product data
- Consent
- Data protection officers
- People's privacy rights

It is important to understand the legal requirements to frame data transfers from the EU to a third country. See, for example, details on the various ways in which data transfer can be done (EU, 2022b).

4.7 Ethics and Informed Consent

According to the EU Commission, "all research proposals that involve the processing of personal data must provide information about the data protection provisions in their proposal." It was also emphasized that

> in principle, living individuals should not be the subject of a research project without being informed, even in the relatively rare cases where research methods, conditions or objectives dictate that they are not made fully aware of the nature of the study until its completion.
>
> *European Commission, 2018*

The European Network of Research Ethics Committees (EUREC) is a network that brings together already existing national Research Ethics Committees (RECs) associations, networks or comparable initiatives at the European level (EUREC, 2022).

The current members represent the following countries (EUREC, 2022):

- Australia
- Belgium
- Czech Republic
- Denmark
- Estonia
- Finland
- France
- Germany
- Greece
- Hungary
- Ireland
- Italy
- Latvia
- Lithuania
- Luxembourg
- Norway
- Portugal
- Slovak Republic (Slovakia)
- Spain
- Sweden
- Switzerland
- The Netherlands

4.8 EU PAS Register®

The European Union's electronic Register of Post-Authorization Studies (EU PAS Register®) is a publicly available register of non-interventional post-authorization studies (PAS) (ENEPP, 2022).

The register has a focus on observational research, which can be applicable to RWE studies, with the purpose of (ENEPP, 2022)

- Increasing transparency
- Reducing publication bias
- Promoting the exchange of information and facilitate collaboration among stakeholders
- Including academia, sponsors and regulatory bodies
- Ensuring compliance with EU pharmacovigilance legislation requirements

4.9 AI

According to the current legislation,

> "artificial intelligence system" (AI system) means software that is developed with one or more of the techniques and approaches listed [below; Annex I of the legislation] and can, for a given set of human-defined objectives, generate outputs such as content, predictions, recommendations, or decisions influencing the environments they interact with.
>
> (EUR-Lex, 2021; European Commission 2022c; European Commission, 2022d)

a. Machine learning approaches, including supervised, unsupervised and reinforcement learning, using a wide variety of methods including deep learning
b. Logic- and knowledge-based approaches, including knowledge representation, inductive (logic) programming, knowledge bases, inference and deductive engines (symbolic) reasoning and expert systems
c. Statistical approaches, Bayesian estimation, search and optimization methods

EU's regulatory framework on AI has the following objectives via a risk-based approach:

- Ensure that AI systems placed on the Union market and used are safe and respect existing law on fundamental rights and Union values
- Ensure legal certainty to facilitate investment and innovation in AI
- Enhance governance and effective enforcement of existing law on fundamental rights and safety requirements applicable to AI systems
- Facilitate the development of a single market for lawful, safe and trustworthy AI applications and prevent market fragmentation.

Remarks

The recent key developments on and emerging trends of RWE to evaluate and enhance patient care were briefly reviewed. Monitoring regulatory guidance documents from multiple regulatory agencies across various jurisdictions that are available were also explained. Relevant topics and standard operating procedures for planning and conduct of post-marketing observational studies must follow the progress on regulatory policies. The data protection impact assessment must also be in place to comply with the GDPR. Finally, actively engaging in relevant public workshops on RWD and RWE held by the EMA and professional societies can help share knowledge and best practices in the big data, RWD and AI space. Finally, since the RWD and RWE landscape is constantly evolving and increasingly playing an important role in medicine and device regulations, it is useful to keep up with the new developments and emerging trends in both the EU and elsewhere.

Disclaimer

Kelly H. Zou is an employee of Viatris. The views expressed are the author's own and do not necessarily represent those of her employer or employers.

References

Arlett, P. DARWIN EU (Data Analytics and Real World Interrogation Network). PCWP and HCPWP Data workshop. September 2020. www.ema.europa.eu/en/documents/presentation/presentation-proposal-darwin-eu-data-analytics-real-world-interrogation-network-parlett-ema_en.pdf (access on March 28. 2022).

Arlett P, Kjaer J, Broich K, Cooke E. Real-World Evidence in EU Medicines Regulation: Enabling Use and Establishing Value. *Clin Pharmacol Ther*. 2022 Jan; 111(1):21–23.

Cave A, Kurz X, Arlett P. Real-World Data for Regulatory Decision Making: Challenges and Possible Solutions for Europe. Clin Pharmacol Ther. 2019 Jul;106(1):36–39.

ENEPP. European Network of Centres for Pharmacoepidemiology and Pharmacovigilance. 2022. www.encepp.eu/index.shtml (access on March 28. 2022).

EUREC. European Network of Research Ethics Committees. 2022. www.eurecnet.org/index.html (access on March 28. 2022).

EUR-Lex, Access to European Union Law. Proposal for a REGULATION OF THE EUROPEAN PARLIAMENT AND OF THE COUNCIL LAYING DOWN HARMONISED RULES ON ARTIFICIAL INTELLIGENCE (ARTIFICIAL INTELLIGENCE ACT) AND AMENDING CERTAIN UNION LEGISLATIVE ACTS. 2021. https://eur-lex.europa.eu/legal-content/EN/TXT/?qid=1623335154975&uri=CELEX%3A52021PC0206 (access on March 28. 2022).

European Commission. Ethics and data protection. 2018. https://ec.europa.eu/info/sites/default/files/5._h2020_ethics_and_data_protection_0.pdf (access on March 28. 2022).

European Commission. A vision for use of real-world evidence in EU medicines regulation. 2021. https://www.ema.europa.eu/en/news/vision-use-real-world-evidence-eu-medicines-regulation (access on March 28. 2022).

European Commission. European Health Data Space. 2022a. https://ec.europa.eu/health/ehealth-digital-health-and-care/european-health-data-space_en (accessed on May 3, 2022).

European Commission. Questions and Answers – EU Health: European Health Data Space (EHDS). 2022b. https://ec.europa.eu/commission/presscorner/detail/en/qanda_22_2712 (accessed on May 3, 2022).

European Commission. Shaping Europe's digital future: big data. 2022c. https://digital-strategy.ec.europa.eu/en/policies/big-data#:~:text=Big%20data%20refers%20to%20large%20amounts%20of%20data,videos%2C%20purchase%20transaction%20records%2C%20GPS%20signals%2C%20and%20more (access on March 28. 2022).

European Commission. A European approach to artificial intelligence. 2022d. https://eur-lex.europa.eu/legal-content/EN/TXT/HTML/?uri=CELEX:52021PC0206&from=EN (access on March 28. 2022).

European Medicines Agency. European medicines agencies network strategy. 2020. www.ema.europa.eu/en/about-us/how-we-work/european-medicines-regulatory-network/european-medicines-agencies-network-strategy#network-strategy-to-2025-section (access on March 28. 2022).

European Medicines Agency. A vision for use of real-world evidence in EU medicines regulation. 2021. www.ema.europa.eu/en/news/vision-use-real-world-evidence-eu-medicines-regulation (access on March 28. 2022).

European Medicines Agency. Initiation of DARWIN EU® Coordination Centre advances integration of real-world evidence into assessment of medicines in the EU. 2022a. www.ema.europa.eu/en/news/initiation-darwin-eur-coordination-centre-advances-integration-real-world-evidence-assessment (access on March 28. 2022).

European Medicines Agency. Data Analysis and Real World Interrogation Network (DARWIN EU). 2022b. www.ema.europa.eu/en/about-us/how-we-work/big-data/data-analysis-real-world-interrogation-network-darwin-eu (access on March 28. 2022).

European Union. Big Data. 2022a. https://digital-strategy.ec.europa.eu/en/policies/big-data (access on March 28. 2022).

European Union. What rules apply if my organisation transfers data outside the EU? 2022b. https://ec.europa.eu/info/law/law-topic/data-protection/reform/rules-business-and-organisations/obligations/what-rules-apply-if-my-organisation-transfers-data-outside-eu_en (access on March 28. 2022).

GDPR.EU. What is GDPR, the EU's new data protection law? 2022. https://gdpr.eu/what-is-gdpr (access on March 28. 2022).

Flynn R, Plueschke K, Quinten C, Strassmann V, Duijnhoven RG, Gordillo-Marañon M, Rueckbeil M, Cohet C, Kurz X. Marketing Authorization Applications Made to the European Medicines Agency in 2018–2019: What was the Contribution of Real-World Evidence? *Clin Pharmacol Ther*. 2022 Jan; 111(1):90–97.

5

Patient Centricity and Precision Medicine

Diana Morgenstern,[1] Mina B. Riad,[1] Claudia Zavala,[1] and Amrit Ray[2]
[1]*Viatris,* [2]*Principled Impact, LLC*

CONTENTS

5.1 Patient Voice

The relationship between real-world data (RWD) and the concept of patient voice is best analyzed by reviewing not only peer-reviewed literature, but also lay press and social media. This combination of sources brings forth valuable information from patients themselves and can lead to more equal communication of insights from medical professionals as well as from those receiving their services (Deloitte, 2018; Smailhodzic et al., 2016; Williamson, 2018). This is particularly important, as the concept of the patient voice seeks to capture what patients themselves want to communicate to the healthcare community at large.

As the healthcare landscape continues to transform, medical affairs professionals are shifting their focus to value-based care (MAPS, 2020). This change requires a refined understanding of what value means to a wide variety of stakeholders, with patients benefiting at the core (McKinsey & Company, 2022). In the current United States (US) landscape of patient-centric healthcare, it is no surprise that a survey of 120 healthcare providers and payers found that 70% of the surveyed organizations see consumer-centric care and patient engagement as a priority. However, according to

DOI: 10.1201/9781003017523-5

Patient Engagement HIT, a network that disseminates the latest information provided by experts on health information technology, this is not being reflected in practice. Patient Engagement HIT reports that payers are only investing an average of 30% of their IT budget in consumer centricity, and healthcare organizations are spending even less at an average of 25%, leading to a lack of innovation and lasting change in this area. Further, only 20% of patients reported any improvements in their healthcare experience in the last few years, as measured by ability to obtain appointments, understand billing information and quality of patient-provider relationships, among other components (Heath, 2017b).

The statistics outlined above suggest a gap between what payers and providers believe will improve patient centricity and what changes patients themselves want to see. Concretely measuring and gathering insights from patients' perspectives could help to narrow this gap if action is taken to incorporate the perspectives into healthcare decision-making. However, implementation of this solution will require both a strong understanding of the patient voice and the ability to convey its value to a wide variety of stakeholders in the healthcare ecosystem (Calvert, O'Connor, & Basch, 2019). To this end, it is crucial to define more thoroughly what is meant by the "patient voice."

Historically, the patient voice consisted mostly of isolated and often-emotional patient anecdotes, but the concept has evolved significantly and now integrates and embraces meaningful, data-driven insights based on patients' perspectives (Pitts, 2019). Today, the patient voice can be more fully understood as opinions and experiences of patients, and how these views inform the medical treatment patients receive (Desouza-Lawrence, 2018). Patients are no longer seen as passive, individualized participants, but active and engaged collective agents in their care (Barry, 2014). As such, the patient voice now provides integral value into healthcare decision-making (Pitts, 2019).

In 2017, a key study by researchers from the National Health Council (NHC; Perfetto et al., 2017) convened a roundtable of 28 organizations (twelve patient organizations, three payers, six professional/policy organizations, five biopharmaceutical organizations, and two research organizations) in order to define components of a patient-centered framework. The organizations, selected through convenience sampling, were asked to describe hallmarks of patient centeredness in the context of patient value in the form of storyboards, illustrative examples, and key themes. Using this information, the NHC then drafted a patient centricity framework rubric which went through a series of iterations informed by the 28 initial organizations, five additional NHC member organizations and three value model developers. The final model yielded components as shown in Table 5.1.

The NHC study outputs can be considered transformative for the concept of patient voice in the current healthcare environment; they provide a tangible framework that can be employed by many stakeholders at large to better gauge the extent of patient voice in their research and interventions.

TABLE 5.1

Components of Patient-centered Framework

Partnership	Patients want to be recognized as integral partners of the development process and are involved in every step of development and dissemination. Examples: patient input is sought at all stages from planning to updating; patient advocacy groups partner with payers to test in practice
Transparency	Assumptions and inputs of an initiative are disclosed to patients in an understandable and timely manner. Examples: project goals are clear and understandable to patients; patients can review drafts/inputs of projects on multiple occasions and through multiple venues
Inclusiveness:	In developing a project, perspectives from a wide variety of stakeholders, including the patient community, are reflected. Examples: projects include a section detailing the importance of seeking and incorporating patient community perspectives; a broad coalition of patient organizations is given the appropriate time to give feedback
Diversity	Differences across patient subpopulations, diseases, life stages, and other factors are accounted for. Examples: studies and other materials for dissemination provide limitations and differences regarding subsections of the target population; models assume the patient population is heterogeneous and take the relevant considerations

Capturing the patient voice can have a wide variety of benefits not only for patients, but for many healthcare stakeholders. For example, research has shown that when patients feel that their voice is being considered, they are more adherent and autonomous, and demonstrate better information recall and higher participation in preventative activities (Desouza-Lawrence, 2018). With regard to clinical research and outcome measurement, including the patient voice allows for a more complete picture of the efficacy of healthcare interventions, because it moves beyond clinical outcomes and highlights patient experiences (Desouza-Lawrence, 2018). For the purposes of improving healthcare practice, insights from the patient voice help pinpoint nuances in patient care, since care is not one-size-fits-all. In the face of many medically reasonable options, it is important to consider each patient's specific characteristics and needs (Barry, 2014). These considerations resonate in the era of precision medicine (PM), which is defined by the National Institute of Health (NIH) as a treatment and prevention method based on the understanding of an individual's genes, environment and lifestyle. As PM seeks to maximize benefits and minimize side effects for the individual, the patient voice becomes important in continuing to capture particularities among patients to further inform healthcare interventions.

How is such an important component of healthcare best captured? There are many qualitative and quantitative measures that can be employed, including patient experience surveys, patient satisfaction surveys, first-hand patient stories gathered from patient advisory groups and councils or focus groups, and RWD collection (Desouza-Lawrence, 2018; Heath, 2017a). RWD can be defined as data collected outside conventional randomized clinical trials (RCTs; McDonald et al., 2019). Within the realm of RWD, researchers can look at electronic health records (EHRs), insurance claims and billing, registries, chart reviews, patient-reported outcomes (PROs), and patient-generated health data (PGHD). PROs reflect how a patient feels and functions at any given point and are collected by surveys. PGHD are typically unstructured data gathered from social media, smart wearables, and similar sources.

In an outcomes-focused environment, RWD is getting increasing attention from more classic investigators due to its ubiquitous nature (McDonald et al., 2019). For example, RWD can be used to complement RCT data since it can be useful in getting information from a much broader population than is reachable via RCTs (Austin, 2020). Conquer Magazine (2020), a publication for cancer patients initiated by the Academy of Oncology Nurse & Patient Navigators that features articles written by and for cancer patients and oncology team members, states "with the use of RWE, effectiveness, patient adherence, long-term patient outcomes, and new safety issues can be revealed for larger numbers of patients." RWD can be used, for example, to promote pharmacovigilance by capturing adverse events that may otherwise be under-reported in clinical trials. Further, artificial intelligence (AI) can be employed to carry out sentiment analysis in large populations, reporting the ratio of positive to negative words used in relation to a drug or treatment to understand how patients are reacting emotionally to the intervention. Additionally, qualitative content analysis can be employed with social media data to answer key questions such as main reasons for switching treatments (McDonald et al., 2019).

Although it has broad appeal, in order to produce meaningful results, RWD must be gathered with a clear objective in mind. When the patient voice is captured through massive data and without a clear goal, insights are harder to glean, clinicians may consider the results to be too generalized, and RWD may not be utilized to effect real change (Coulter et al., 2014). With that in mind, it is crucial to include patients when determining the process for capturing input. A recent literature review of peer-reviewed publications that employed PROs in cancer clinical studies found that much of the time, the potential of PROs was not fully realized, with researchers using insufficient measures to gather data, using measures that did not fit best with the study, or failing to correctly disseminate findings to patients (Addario et al., 2019). Given these findings, the authors proposed that studies include patients from the beginning of the research process by asking them what outcomes would be meaningful, how they want these outcomes to be captured, including input on choice of language, and how the key insights should be disseminated within patient communities.

Ultimately, three key components must be in place for RWD to be correctly leveraged (Austin, 2020). First, there must be a clear focus on value, defined as how the data gathered will hold patient-centered care at its core. Second, there must be "actionability", defined as having a plan to incorporate key insights into tangible clinical decision-making. Third, technology alignment, that is to say access to the appropriate technological resources to support data gathering, must be considered.

Several examples illustrate the use of RWD to help capture the patient voice. In cancer research, PROs such as progression-free survival, overall survival, and toxicities can be gathered to complement data from clinical trials and get a more complete picture of how patients respond to treatment (Klink, 2020). Noona, a smart cloud-based mobile service, allows oncology patients to report real-time symptoms and lets their healthcare providers access that information in order to better recognize early warning signs and send tailored self-care instructions, schedule a clinic visit, or evaluate possible treatment changes (Conquer Magazine, 2020). HealthTree is a software tool that allows multiple myeloma patients to enter their information into a large patient network (Conquer Magazine, 2020). This tool was developed based on the finding that electronic health records only capture about 8% of patients' complete data, leading to a gap in relevant information collected. As such, HealthTree makes a point of collecting data regarding questions not typically captured by health care providers (HCPs), such as, "What can you do on your own?" "Do you have an autoimmune disorder?" and "Do you have quality- of-life issues?" The responses give researchers access to ample information that may help them to answer scientific questions in ways that cannot be tackled by oncology clinical trials.

RWD has also been utilized to discern patient voice in other noncommunicable diseases (NCDs). Veradigm, for example, a health information technology, analytics and intervention solutions company, has employed Natural Language Processing to analyze its cloud-based electronic health records to understand patients with type 2 diabetes and cardiovascular and/or renal comorbidities (Farah et al., 2022). Using de-identified data from their large, cloud-based, bi-directional EHR platform for ambulatory patients in the US, researchers studied the impact of these comorbidities on patient responsiveness to select glucose-lowering treatments.

Finally, Inspire, a social network for health that connects patients and caregivers worldwide to share experiences and express support via medical condition communities (Inspire, 2020), employed linguistic analysis of social media text to understand ways in which patients communicate about chronic pain (Inspire, 2019). The researchers utilized natural language processing (NLP) to mine large unstructured texts (over 4 million posts), along with iterative hands-on linguistic analysis. This analysis yielded insights such as the value that chronic pain patients place on using language that validates their pain even when the pain may not be perceivable, the wide use of metaphors to convey diverse experiences of pain, and utilization of the "spoonie" social identity to promote social ties within the chronic pain community. Findings such as these furnish essential patient voice and help provide perspective and refinement to our understanding of "unmet" medical needs.

5.2 Patient Journey Mapping

Patient journey mapping (PJM) is a holistic view of all touchpoints or interactions between a patient and the healthcare system. It enables a view from the patient's perspective, which may identify critical points of services that need improvement. It allows researchers to understand and visualize the patient's experiences physically, emotionally and clinically, thus, aiding in finding solutions and ways to ease the patient journey. The goal of PJM is to provide a visual representation of every interaction a patient might have with the medical community in order to improve the patient's satisfaction along each step of their care, to keep the patient engaged, adherent to therapy and enhance the chances of a successful outcome (Trebble et al. 2010). Thus, the journey can typically be longitudinal over time.

For individual patients, the ease of their specific journeys through healthcare encounters is a key to successful outcomes. If patients are not well-informed of the aspects of their healthcare journey and are not well engaged in the entire process, this may lead to poor outcomes or rejections of care. For example, a potential consequence would be non- or low adherence.

More broadly speaking, PJM can be developed based on RWD to inform various aspects of decision-making and can then be examined for key decision points (i.e., encounters or interactions). The process might be improved to allow for efficient care and a satisfactory experience for the patient. Process-analysis can help test mutiple scenarios in decision-making to identify key opportunities for improvement. The success of PJM depends upon the encounters, interactions, process details, actionable insights, and alignment across providers on the goals for care.

In terms of NCDs, the PJM process ultimately describes how a person receiving healthcare manages an acute or chronic condition (e.g., a theoretical framework depicting the common touchpoints along the patient journey for NCDs in low- and middle- income countries [LMICs]; Devi et al., 2020). A successful PJM identifies the critical moments that have the potential to influence patients, healthcare professionals and other stakeholders in order to assure successful movement along the identified care pathway.

PJM describes the stages of patient care, beginning with the onset of symptoms, through diagnosis and therapy, and ending with either recovery and optimizing treatment or adjustment to a new lifestyle. Figure 5.1 shows a

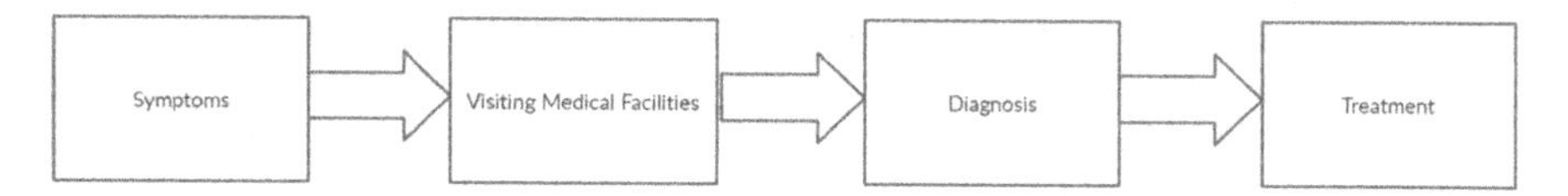

FIGURE 5.1
Patient journey.

hypothetical patient's perspective of the steps he or she goes through. Within each step, a comprehensive map brings to life gaps, bottlenecks and other potential issues along the course of events. Herein, we only discuss obstacles that the patient may face in a simple map.

Symptoms are typically the first experience of illness for a patient. Some patients may immediately seek medical assessments even with mild symptoms, some may wait for their annual physical, and some not recognize, neglect, deny, or decide to accept symptoms without any further actions. This first step of PJM allows researchers to identify obstacles from the patient side and how their emotional experiences can affect their approach to health. In the case of NCDs, the earlier a patient takes an action (e.g., visiting an HCP) after experiencing the first sign of a symptom, the faster the patient can mover to diagnosis, management and control of the disease. For example, the earlier the discovery of cancer, the greater the chance is for successful prognosis and therapy. Management of the patient's discovery step can be supported by utilizing tools like electronic PROs, questionnaires, surveys, or diagnostic modalities both outside or inside a medical facility (Hackett and Cassem 1969).

Visiting an HCP is an important step in PJM. This touchpoint or encounter can provide useful information about the patient's experience at the enoucnter (e.g., office visit, emergency department visit, and intensive care unit stay). Moreover, the element of "time" impacts the patient's journey. The patient must make an appointment, which may result in a time lag to receiving service, during which the condition may worsen. When the appointment arrives, however, the amount of time a patient spends in the HCP's office and the number of providers she or he interacts with will also impact the journey (Klassen and Yoogalingam 2013). Multiple appointments may be necessary to arrive at an accurate diagnosis. The communication between the HCP and the patient must be clear, despite complicated medical terminology that the patient may find difficult to comprehend. By mapping this step and considering all the problems the patient may face with, medical staff can work to eliminate unnecessary burdens and give the patient better experience along the way.

Diagnoses may not be straightforward at first, and thus, the HCP may ask for further workups such as lab tests or refer the patient to a specialist for further evaluations. Once the diagnosis more certain, the patient can experience anxiety, distress, or fear, especially for life-threatening or uncurable diseases, for example, these phenoma can be common during the coronavirus disease 2019 (COVID-19) pandemic. Communicating the diagnosis to the patient must be forthcoming, considerate, and ethical. There are protocols for delivering the "bad" news or diagnosis, e.g., SPIKES (a six-step protocol for delivering bad news) (BUtOW et al. 1996). Some diseases require a change in a patient's lifestyle and a clear discussion of the different treatment options with the patient and caregivers, especially since questions may arise regarding the diagnosis, treatment options, and prognosis. Mapping these steps can provide a better understanding of patient's emotional and physical reactions and the following actions..

Treatments can be challenging for some patients, for example, treatments requiring chronic administration or a long-term commitment. Obtaining medication records may present many obstacles since medications using RWD may not be easy since a patient may not have health insurance coverage or a medication may require prior authorizations. A high deductible and a lack of insurance also create out-of-pocket (OOP) cost burden (Kesselheim, Avorn and Sarpatwari, 2016).

In settings like retail pharmacies or emergency departments, the likelihood of recording or billing errors increases. For example, diagnosis codes, medication class, prescription directions, quantity prescribed, medication fills and refills can all be subject to errors (Cheung, Bouvy and De Smet 2009, Yang et al. 2018, Gregory et al. 2021). At a pharmacy, the consultation time between the pharmacist and the patient may be non-existent to brief, depending upon a multitude of factors. Consultation with a pharmacist is critical and beneficial for some prescriptions which have complicated instructions. PJM can identify the areas where improvement is needed in the training of healthcare providers, as well as new opportunities to improve patient interactions and educating by providing simple pictorial representations to patients (Hogan 2011).

Healthcare process-mapping also facilitates record-audit purposes by documenting how patient journeys are monitored and managed, e.g., via good clinical practice, cost efficiencies and the patient's personal satisfaction. In order to improve a patient's satisfaction with the healthcare system, stakeholders must be engaged and aligned to optimize and maximize care.

The analysis of RWD can allow the healthcare ecosystem to identify deficiencies and gaps. An in-depth review of how the medical community interacts with patients and what the outcomes are following the touchpoints are critical for improving the quality and efficiency of patient care. .

PJM can identify and characterize both the valuable and unnessary steps along a patient's journey. Analysis can then lead to redesign of the care pathway to enhance value-added steps but remove non- or low-value-added ones. Periodic reviews of a patient's journey can be beneficialfor continuous improvement throughout the entire patient experience (McCarthy et al. 2016).

Overall, there are several advantages of PJM, with the patient experience as the focus of the mapping process:

- Streamlining activities to comply with regulations
- Refining HCPs' duties
- Eliminate systematic waste
- Reducing unwanted or unnecessary costs
- Ehancing patient's and caregivers' experience
- Increasing the awareness and understanding of the disease, comorbidities, and trajectaries

To identify the right patient, right medicine at the right time, PM is an approach to the prevention and treatment of disease in an individual patient that takes into consideration the unique influence of genetic, environmental and lifestyle factors (Ray et al., 2019). While its use remains limited, PM is not a new concept in clinical medicine, e.g., a person receiving a blood transfusion is not randomly given another's blood. Bioinformatics involves the integration of computers, software tools, and databases to address biological questions. These approaches are often used for major initiatives that generate RWD. The exponential growth of data-availability (e.g., digital therapeutics and apps) that considers a person's uniqueness that confers susceptibility to an illness or benefit from a particular treatment. With PM, treatments are designed for that unique individual.

Final Remarks

In summary, PJM, patient voice, medicine, as well as personalized medicines are useful concepts, and data-driven decisions may be made through these applications.

As evidenced by the information outlined throughtout this chapter, the patient voice and RWD are entwined, both conceptually and practically. The utilization of innovative sources of data such as PROs and RWD can help to ensure that the patient voice truly captures patients' needs and experiences, helping to accurately reflect how healthcare interventions are impacting patients in their natural environment. Complementing traditional approaches, such as RCTs, with these innovative measures to elaborate a complete picture of the patient voice, can lead to more meaningful and successful outcomes for patients, providers and payers alike.

Disclaimer

Diana Morgenstern is a former employee of Upjohn, a Division of Pfizer, and Viatris. Mina B. Riad and Claudia Zavala are former contractors of Upjohn, a Division of Pfizer, and Viatris. Amrit Ray is an employee of Principled Impact, LLC and a former employee of Upjohn, a Division of Pfizer, and Viatris. The views expressed are the authors' own and do not necessarily represent those of the employer. The authors appreciate the editorial support from Arghya Bhattacharya and Aswin Kumar A of Viatris.

References

Addario B, Geissler J, Horn MK, Krebs LU, Maskens D, Oliver K, Plate A, Schwartz E, Willmarth N. Including the patient voice in the development and implementation of patient-reported outcomes in cancer clinical trials. Health Expect. 2020 Feb;23(1):41–51.

Austin E, LeRouge C, Hartzler AL, Segal C, Lavallee DC. Capturing the patient voice: implementing patient-reported outcomes across the health system. Qual Life Res. 2020 Feb;29(2):347–355.

Barry, M. Giving Patients a Voice in Care Decisions.2014. https://qioprogram.org/qionews/articles/giving-patients-voice-care-decisions (Accessed on March 30, 2022).

Butow PN, Kazemi JN, Beeney LJ, Griffin AM, Dunn SM, Tattersall MH. When the diagnosis is cancer: patient communication experiences and preferences. Cancer. 1996 Jun 15;77(12):2630–7.

Calvert MJ, O'Connor DJ, Basch EM. Harnessing the patient voice in real-world evidence: the essential role of patient-reported outcomes. Nat Rev Drug Discov. 2019 Sep;18(10):731–732.

Cheung KC, Bouvy ML, De Smet PA. Medication errors: the importance of safe dispensing. Br J Clin Pharmacol. 2009 Jun;67(6):676–80.

Conquer: The Patient Voice. From Real-World Evidence to Real-World Outcomes: How Real-World Patients Are Changing the Treatment of Multiple Myeloma. 2020. https://conquer-magazine.com/issues/special-issues/april-2020-how-real-world-evidence-has-the-potential-to-shape-real-world-outcomes (Accessed on March 30, 2022).

Coulter A, Locock L, Ziebland S, Calabrese J. Collecting data on patient experience is not enough: they must be used to improve care. BMJ. 2014 Mar 26;348:g2225.

Deloitte. 2018 Global health care outlook: the evolution of smart care. 2018. www2.deloitte.com/content/dam/Deloitte/global/Documents/Life-Sciences-Health-Care/gx-lshc-hc-outlook-2018.pdf (Accessed on March 30, 2022).

Desouza-Lawrence, D. What is Patient Voice and Why Does it Matter? Jayex. 2018. www.jayex.com/en-au/blog/why-patient-voice-is-key-to-improving-patient-engagement (Accessed on March 30, 2022).

Devi R, Kanitkar K, Narendhar R, Sehmi K, Subramaniam K. A Narrative Review of the Patient Journey Through the Lens of Non-communicable Diseases in Low- and Middle-Income Countries. Adv Ther. 2020 Dec;37(12):4808–4830.

Gregory H, Cantley M, Calhoun C, Hall GA, Matuskowitz AJ, Weant KA. Incidence of prescription errors in patients discharged from the emergency department. Am J Emerg Med. 2021 Aug;46:266–270.

Hackett TP, Cassem NH. Factors contributing to delay in responding to the signs and symptoms of acute myocardial infarction. Am J Cardiol. 1969 Nov;24(5):651–8.

Heath, S. How to Integrate the Patient Voice into Healthcare Decision-Making. Patient Engagement Hit. 2017a. https://patientengagementhit.com/news/how-to-integrate-the-patient-voice-into-healthcare-decision-making (Accessed on March 30, 2022).

Heath, S. Patient, Provider Views Diverge on Consumer Centric Care Priority. Patient Engagement Hit. 2017b. https://patientengagementhit.com/news/patient-provider-views-diverge-on-consumer-centric-care-priority (Accessed on March 30, 2022).

Hogan, M.E. Enhancing medication adherence by improving the clarity of labels for prescription drugs. Canadian Pharmacists Journal/Revue des Pharmaciens du Canada, 2011; 144(5):236–239.

Inspire. Linguistic Analysis and Audience Insights: How Chronic Pain Patients Communicate About Pain. 2019. https://corp.inspire.com/resource/chronic-pain-audience-insights (Accessed on March 30, 2022).

Inspire. Our story. 2020. https://corp.inspire.com/meet-inspire/our-story/. (Accessed on March 30, 2022).

Kesselheim AS, Avorn J, Sarpatwari A. The High Cost of Prescription Drugs in the United States: Origins and Prospects for Reform. JAMA. 2016 Aug 23–30;316(8):858–71.

Klassen, K.J., & Yoogalingam, R. Appointment system design with interruptions and physician lateness. International Journal of Operations & Production Management. 2013. www.emerald.com/insight/content/doi/10.1108/01443571311307253/full/html (Accessed on March 30, 2022).

Klink, A. Incorporating the patient voice in real-world evidence for healthcare stakeholders. Focus Magazine. 2020. www.cardinalhealth.com/en/services/manufacturer/biopharmaceutical/real-world-evidence-and-insights/resources-for-real-world-evidence-and-insights/focus-magazine/patient-voice-in-real-world-evidence-for-healthcare-stakeholders.html# (Accessed on March 30, 2022).

McCarthy, S., O'Raghallaigh, P., Woodworth, S., Lim, Y.L., Kenny, L.C. & Adam, F. An integrated patient journey mapping tool for embedding quality in healthcare service reform. J Decision Syst., 2016; *25*(sup1): 354–368.

McDonald L, Malcolm B, Ramagopalan S, Syrad H. Real-world data and the patient perspective: the PROmise of social media? BMC Med. 2019 Jan 16;17(1):11.

McKinsey & Company. The next frontier of care delivery in healthcare. 2022. www.mckinsey.com/industries/healthcare-systems-and-services/our-insights/the-next-frontier-of-care-delivery-in-healthcare (Accessed on March 30, 2022).

Medical Affairs Professional Society. Communicating the Value of Medical Affairs: A MAPS White Paper. MAPS. 2020. https://medicalaffairs.org/wp-content/uploads/2020/08/MAPS-White-Paper_Comm-Value-of-Medical-Affairs_May20201.pdf (Accessed on March 30, 2022).

Perfetto EM, Oehrlein EM, Boutin M, Reid S, Gascho E. Value to Whom? The Patient Voice in the Value Discussion. Value Health. 2017 Feb;20(2):286–291.

Pitts PJ. Towards Meaningful Engagement for the Patient Voice. Patient. 2019 Aug;12(4):361–363.

Ray A, Zou KH, Ewing S. Real world evidence for precision medicine. CIO Applications. 2019. www.cioapplications.com/cxoinsights/real-world-evidence-for-precision-medicine-nid-4676.html (Accesed on March 30, 2022).

Smailhodzic E, Hooijsma W, Boonstra A, Langley DJ. Social media use in healthcare: A systematic review of effects on patients and on their relationship with healthcare professionals. BMC Health Serv Res. 2016 Aug 26;16(1):442.

Trebble TM, Hansi N, Hydes T, Smith MA, Baker M. Process mapping the patient journey: an introduction. BMJ. 2010 Aug 13;341:c4078.

Yeoman G, Furlong P, Seres M, Binder H, Chung H, Garzya V, Jones RR. Defining patient centricity with patients for patients and caregivers: a collaborative endeavour. BMJ Innov. 2017 Apr;3(2):76–83.

Farah J, Wilk A, Nguyen N, Vasey J, Kallenbach Lee. Type 2 Diabetes and Management of Cardiovascular and Renal Comorbidities: A Cohort Analysis with Case Study Using Electronic Health Records. Veradigm. 2022. https://veradigm.com/img/resource-comorbidities-type-2-diabetes-rwe.pdf (Accessed on March 30, 2022).

Williamson C. Combining professional and lay knowledge to improve patient care. Br J Gen Pract. 2018 Jan;68(666):39–40.

Yang Y, Ward-Charlerie S, Dhavle AA, Rupp MT, Green J. Quality and Variability of Patient Directions in Electronic Prescriptions in the Ambulatory Care Setting. J Manag Care Spec Pharm. 2018 Jul;24(7):691–699.

Yeoman G, Furlong P, Seres M, Binder H, Chung H, Garzya V, Jones RR. Defining patient centricity with patients for patients and caregivers: a collaborative endeavour. BMJ Innov. 2017 Apr;3(2):76–83.

6

Health Information Technology

Joseph P. Cook, Gabriel Jipa, Claudia Zavata, and Lobna A. Salem
Viatris

CONTENTS

6.1 Contemporary eHealth

The digital age has continued to provide new technologies to support access to quality healthcare. This fundamental digitization has been applied to healthcare in a number of ways and for separable purposes. While electronic healthcare (eHealth) covers the whole range of electronic technologies applied to healthcare, principally related to computing, mobile health (mHealth) relates to that subset that uses mobile technologies that share information over the radio waves. mHealth has been described as having a broader scope, including patient education, health promotion, disease self-management, healthcare cost savings, and remote monitoring—while telemedicine focuses on the elements of diagnosis and treatment (Bali et al., 2018). All these efforts be used to support improvements in patient care, and for our purposes, we will consider both in the overview provided here.

First, we may use these technologies to measure outcomes in real time with continuously recorded data, these can be via responsive survey requests or

DOI: 10.1201/9781003017523-6

through routine processes or timing. Second, we may try to motivate patients to improve adherence and improve their health and the effectiveness of the healthcare system. Combined with data recording, there is a means of testing alternative approaches to improving adherence and leveraging the results. Third, we can have improved patient connectivity with the healthcare provider or system provides the potential for better response time can be used to enhance the patient experience and make the treatment pathway more efficient. Finally, if shared and leveraged appropriately, these richer and more timely recordings of patient experiences can enhance pharmacovigilance efforts as well as efforts to better define the best treatment pathway for patients and perhaps alternative treatment pathways for appropriately defined subpopulations.

Before moving on, let us consider the underlying broader array of new technology that we build on in healthcare for eHealth and mHealth. Today, with a world population of about 7.6 billion, The International Telecommunication Union's (ITU) data indicate that more than half of the world is connected to the Internet and there are more than 8 billion mobile telephone subscriptions worldwide. The subscriptions exceed the population as some people have more than one, and some people do not have a mobile phone. In the US, the figures for computer and internet use are estimated to be well over half the population and closer to 80 percent as of 2015 (US Census Bureau, 2015). Reports by the Pew Trust had internet use at about 90 percent and mobile telephony up to 95 percent by 2018 (Pew Research Center).

Mobile telephony continues to expand the digital reach well beyond the network of copper wires. An implication of these new technology companies and their reach into the economy and society is their potential to transform healthcare and healthcare markets. Apple's user base, as of 2016, was 85.8 million iPhone owners worldwide and more than 13 million just in the US alone. Compare that figure with one of the US's largest insurers, United Healthcare as an insurance carrier and payer, with about 50 million enrollees in its health insurance offerings. Such a large technology-based footprint no doubt helped Apple to recruit 400,000 people in less than a year for its Apple Watch heart health study with Stanford University, in an era of significant recruitment challenges (Christina Farr, 2019). Digital devices, personal computers, and microprocessors are increasingly ubiquitous in our daily lives. Microprocessors appear now not only in every sort of product from refrigerators to automobiles, but also in a range of medical products, including blood pressure monitors, spirometers (lung capacity), pulse oximeters and heart rate monitors, magnetic resonance (MR) imaging and computed tomography (CT) scanners, sonograph or ultrasound machines, defibrillators, digital flow sensors, fetal heart monitors, and, of course, wearables (Verdict, 2020). Most are embedded devices that tacitly transmit the resulting data into a computer system for storage and review by healthcare providers.

The impact of telemedicine is particularly high in rural settings, where access issues are more acutely felt. A lack of local healthcare resources only enhances the opportunity for improvements exploiting the rapid expansion of mobile and internet access. Population health can be enhanced by the expanded reach of telemedicine with eHealth, particularly mHealth. Both health literacy and expert medical advice are poised to have greater reach than ever before. Moreover, health profession education in the more rural and developing parts of the world could also be augmented (Strasser and Regaldo, 2016).

The response to coronavirus disease 2019 (COVID-19) has included the expansions of various elements of healthcare access for patients, including access to telemedicine and providing a case study that will no doubt be studied for insights for years to come. Several steps were taken at the federal level and were cognizant of the connection between COVID-19 and chronic conditions, many noncommunicable diseases (NCDs), that can act as risk factors for the disease. The Families First Coronavirus Response Act in the US mandated that all insurance plans—Medicare, Medicaid, military, Affordable Care Act (ACA), and employer—cover the cost of a coronavirus test, roughly $50, and any related doctor's appointment copays or fees (CMS, 2020a). Further, the Centers for Medicare & Medicaid Services (CMS, 2020b) has expanded federal access to allow prescription fills of covered Part D drugs—including insulin—for up to a three-month supply; flexibility for more medication delivery options—such as mail or home delivery through retail pharmacies; expanding telehealth to maintain access to doctors.

Private insurers took similar steps with respect to other chronic conditions by working with manufacturers to arrange discounts that directly impacted patients out of pocket (OOP) costs. This extended to a wide range of products beyond the reduction for insulin under the federal mandate. Moreover, the federal tax authorities also expanded the definition of "preventative" care to include care for some chronic conditions as well, while still qualifying for use of tax-advantaged healthcare savings accounts that were designed as companions for the increasingly widely used high deductible plans.

As with the US federal government's insurance plans, private plans also altered conditions to improve access to allow home delivery of prescriptions by local pharmacies, as well as delivery via mail order. Prescriptions every 90 days, instead of the common 30-day prescriptions, reduced the interactions with the pharmacy to maintain adequate supplies of their medications. Perhaps most importantly, they offered greater access to telemedicine and remote counseling. These expansions to access included expanded telemedicine access, particularly in the form of coverage for "audio only" visits, which has been a source of some tension in the past (American College of Obstetricians and Gynecologists, press release June 26, 2020).

Historically, stakeholders have expressed their concerns over the use of telemedicine or took action to restrict its broader use. For example, the

Federation of State Medical Boards (FSMB, 2014) adopted a definition of telemedince that would generally exclude "an audio-only, telephone conversation, e-mail/instant messaging conversation or fax". The position was subsequently explained, although not intended to limit use of the telephone, to protect patient safety and prevent care being limited for extended periods to that based on audio only (Gillespie, 2014). The concerns over audio only also extend to costs. For example, a few years ago, the Massachusetts Hospital Association organized a coalition to support a bill that would require parity of payment between in office and virtual visits, while the Massachusetts Association of Health Plans (representing 17 private plans) argued that allowing a phone call to be billed at the rate of an office visit would do little to create cost saving efficiencies in the system (Bailey, 2016). This example illustrates the more general tension between technology creating new opportunities for care and the system needing to learn through a market process how to price them at efficient levels; however, it is worth noting that, in more recent responses to COVID-19, the FSMB reported on a number of states including "audio-only" within the definition of reimbursable telemedicine explicitly (FSMB, 2022).

There is evidence that patient preferences for telemedicine seems stronger for younger patients and, quite sensibly, for patients with further to travel for care. Similarly, being a frequent user of care is also predictive of a preference for seeking care via telemedicine (Mehrotra et al., 2013). Patient satisfaction seems relatively high for many patients, as well. Eighty-five percent of patients gave their physicians the highest rating on a 5-point scale in 28,222 encounters between 24,040 patients and 277 physicians between January 2013 and August 2016 (Martinez et al., 2018). Most commonly, these encounters were with family medicine physicians and indicated an urgent care retail clinic would have been the alternative. Less commonly, about one quarter of the time, patients used a coupon. Coupons use and the receipt of a prescription were positively correlated with high satisfaction scores.

As patients seem receptive to telemedicine and indications are that a portion of their care can be satisfactorily provided in this way, these expansions may hold and allow for greater use of an ever-growing tranche of technologies. However, for this to truly stick, overuse will have to be avoided and the economics will have to work for insurers and other stakeholders. As these technologies are more widely used, the available data from which to develop evidence will continue to expand and become ever more valuable. For example, one estimate put the growth in the size of digital universe to be more than 100-fold, growing from 130 exabytes in 2005 to about 16,000 exabytes in 2017 (Dash et al., 2019). Moreover, these technologies will also serve to deliver back care with lower transactions costs and even, perhaps, therapeutic effect.

A variety of digital or "smart" packaging options have been developed to help address the problem of patients' medication adherence (Forcinio, 2017).

Some medicines can be distributed in a wireless pill bottle that can sense and record being opened or closed and a measure of the contents. It can also send a signal by computer to the physician and patient if a dose appears to have been missed; the bottle can also emit a flash or tone for the same purpose. Or the cap may also track the time between openings of the bottle to help keep patients' medication schedule on track. Data from devices such as these can also, when transmitted into a healthcare system, provide additional data for discernment of and evidence for improved treatment regimens based on RWD.

The interplay between technology as a source of collecting data and a means of improving healthcare knowledge management to aid healthcare providers, as well as a tool to improve outcomes and develop the most current evidence of effects is strong. Perhaps one of the closest relationships is in electronic devices and digital platforms that both keep track of the patient's adherence and progress, but also serve as a means of treatment. The "gamification" of healthcare reached a milestone with the Food & Drug Administration's (FDA) approval EndeavorRx as a prescription only treatment for children with attention deficit hyperactivity disorder (ADHD). This was the first time the FDA had permitted marketing of a game-based digital therapeutic (DTx) device. With such advances, we may see the lines blur between approaches across functions, including data collection for analysis, population-based assessments of evidence of efficacy, and treatment.

6.2 Artificial Intelligence

During the last decade, we have seen the incredible growth and innovation in technology, including artificial intelligence (AI), due to incredible increases in availability of digital data, more powerful and high-performance computing, and breakthroughs in machine learning (ML) research. AI, sometimes called machine intelligence, refers to the ability of a machine (or process) to respond to environmental stimuli or data, modify its operations based on this new information, and maximize performance (Benke & Benke, 2018). AI techniques have become an essential part of the technology industry, helping to solve many challenging problems in computer science, software engineering and operations research. Within the healthcare space, AI innovations can assist physician decision making, unlock powerful medical insights, free up time for healthcare professionals to prioritize the most in-need patients, and more.

There are 703 million people who are aged 65 or older, and the projected count will be 1.5 billion by 2050. The UN has estimated that 1 in 6 people in the world will be over the age 65 by 2050, up from 1 in 11 in 2019 (UN DESA,

2021). The rise of NCDs has been driven by primarily four major risk factors: tobacco use, physical inactivity, the harmful use of alcohol and unhealthy diets (WHO, 2022). In light of these changes, it comes as no surprise that the demand for healthcare will continue to grow exponentially, leading to a shortage of about 13 million health care providers (HCPs) by 2035 (WHO) and potential issues in terms of financial sustainability (McKinsey & Co., 2020). In conjunction with these challenges, it is relevant to state that the healthcare landscape is changing from a commercial-based model to a value- and evidence-based model (Werner et al., 2021). These and other challenges can be tackled with the assistive power of AI.

Within the broad scope of AI, there are several key technologies that are taking center stage, especially in relation to healthcare (Mindfields, 2018). For instance, Natural Language Processing (NLP) entails taking unstructured data such as electronic health records (EHRs), clinical notes, journal articles, and other valuable information that may not be linked, and creating meaning out of it by highlighting relevant information. NLP allows for this to be done quickly and seamlessly, where it would take several HCPs many hours to tie all of this information together and pinpoint the links between the data. Another important technology within AI is deep learning (DL). This entails training a machine with previously available information until the model is "locked", and the machine can then utilize these complex algorithms to perform tasks like diagnosis, prediction, and treatment selection. Thirdly, Context Aware Processing (CAP) can help create efficient chatbots to greatly reduce the burden of HCPs in responding to all patients in real time. They can be used to direct patients to the right HCP and even provide accurate solutions to simple problems. Finally, intelligent robotics can be used in developing tools for surgical procedures, or in developing companions for those suffering from mental illness of cognitive decay due to lack of interaction with others.

Importantly, the American Hospital Association (2019) highlights four key building blocks of effective AI application for healthcare: people, policies, resources and technology. People refer to the responsibility of individuals to lead, oversee, and use AI systems. Although these technologies may appear to "think" for themselves, they still require responsible experts to employ them and make the ultimate decisions. Policies refer to the regulatory and ethical frameworks that need to be in place in regard to data access and patient security, as AI runs on data from various information systems. Resources refers to supporting the AI team with a strong operating budget to ensure HCPs have the needed training, planning, and testing for the AI to be used in the smoothest way possible. Finally, technology refers to the need to invest in the most appropriate technologies depending on the institutions' goals and priorities, generating the most effective insights possible.

When looking at these technologies, we can see how AI today is able to uncover powerful insights through pattern recognition with flexibility and ease. It should be noted that this is a great improvement from the AI of yesterday, which was limited to rules-based behavior and automation. We can expect that the AI of the future will become increasingly context-based, more complex, and become more and more similar to human intelligence (Booz Allen Hamilton Inc., 2022). Currently, AI's role in healthcare can be leveraged in a variety of points along the continuum of care, such as prevention, diagnosis, treatment, and follow-up. For the purposes of this chapter, we will now focus on three key areas of utility: diagnosis, clinical trials, and unstructured data cleaning.

Since diseases such as NCDs and health threats such as communicable diseases, including viruses, are constantly evolving, the healthcare industry is one that requires fast-paced innovation and adaptation. In this sense, AI's role in early diagnosis holds tremendous promise. As McKinsey (2020) mentions, many medical specialties naturally benefit from these technologies, such as radiology, pathology, dermatology, and ophthalmology. In these areas, detecting subtle patterns or finding small markers can be a time-consuming and laborious task for HCPs to undertake. Therefore, AI technologies can help significantly increase productivity, expedite life-saving decisions, and lessen time to diagnosis while lowering costs.

According to the American Hospital Association (2019), AI is trained to diagnose by first learning from thousands of real-life examples—comparing patients' symptoms against known disease states—until they learn to spot patterns and identify links between symptoms and illnesses. Then, AI can draw conclusions in less than a second, prioritize and order the most relevant test a patient might need in real time, identify the most at-risk patients for closer monitoring, and expedite image interpretation for a quicker result. Importantly, a meta-analysis of 25 clinical studies found that AI (in particular, DL) is able to diagnose with the same percentage of accuracy as health care professioanls (Liu et al., 2019). Although the authors call for more studies, these promising findings illustrate the potential of AI to aid HCPs in diagnosis without compromising accuracy.

Several examples can be used to further illustrate this point. For instance, doctors aided by Google developed a complex algorithm for detecting risk of cardiovascular illness by training a system to recognize patterns in retinal images. Through ML, this system was able to analyze over 280,000 already existing images of patients and then predict which new patients were at risk for cardiovascular complications based on blood vessel abnormalities (Kashyap, 2018). In another case, a study showed that a technology using DL networks proved to be superior to a group of dermatologists in diagnosing skin cancer. While human HCPs caught 86.6% of cases, the AI caught 95% (Haenssle et al., 2018). This was both because the AI missed fewer melanomas (meaning it had higher sensitivity) and misdiagnosed fewer benign moles as malignant (which means it had higher specificity). The implications are clear: more patients will be correctly diagnosed and less patients will undergo unnecessary tests or treatment.

Another important example is that of software created by scientists through ML at Imperial College London. This technology was able to identify and measure the severity of small vessel disease through analyzing CT scans with a learned mechanism, helping HCPs to administer best treatment quickly and accurately to patients at risk of stroke and dementia (Chen et al., 2018). This new method has the ability to improve diagnosis beyond the abilities of the human eye, provide insight in emergency decision-making, and allow for monitoring of dementia. ML has also been applied in diagnosing fibromyalgia. One system called FM-pain was able to identify, through ML, and fMRI-based neurological signature for physical fibromyalgia-related pain (López-Sola et al., 2017). This can help not only with faster diagnoses, but also in characterizing how and where patients' pain is linked to their brain, promoting more targeted treatment and interventions. In the area of mental health, one study tested an Embodied Conversational Agent's ability to diagnose major depressive disorder (MDD) through a clinical interview and found that this tool is an effective way to conduct an empathetic assessment, reaching a sensitivity of 73% and specificity of 95% (Philip et al., 2018). This encouraging finding demonstrates that software such as ECAs have the ability to take on the diagnosis process, freeing up time and resources for mental health professionals to spend on psychotherapy.

Turning now to patients who is the center of healthcare, the role of AI in diagnostics also has various positive implications in terms of empowering patients to take charge of their own health. As stated by McKinsey (2020), currently the only way patients have of knowing if they need to see a doctor is to see one—and that needs to change. Patients are demanding answers more quickly, and there is a growing call for patient empowerment. AI can help in this regard by allowing patients to monitor and take charge of their own health through home monitoring, self-care, and community-based care. This falls in line with the changing healthcare landscape, leaning towards patient centricity, and with the changing global trends, which portend an increase in chronic conditions. For example, patients with diabetes, previously encouraged to monitor their symptoms by continuous hospital visits, can now self-monitor at home through AI-enabled blood glucose monitoring devices. This can also be leveraged in emergency room scenarios, with AI-based apps, such as Babylon or Mediktor enabling e-triage, to potentially reduce clinical workload of HCPs (McKinsey, 2020). As can be seen through these examples, AI has unprecedented potential in faster and more accurate diagnoses, which has positive implications for patients, doctors, and the healthcare system at large.

Randomized controlled trials (RCTs) are a key part of the process of getting medicines safely from the lab to the market. As important as they are, traditional RCTs have some gaps to improve upon; in particular, patient recruitment and accrual speed. Studies show that it takes an average of 15 years to bring a drug to market, and one third of this time is spent on patient recruitment since the cohort composition needs to representatively reflect the larger population (Harrer et al., 2019). This results in a lengthy process with only a 10% success rate. Turning to the financial aspect, patient recruitment is necessary to ensure trial efficacy but takes up 32% of economic resources in the clinical trial process. This results in a significant burden since it is often challenging to recruit suitable patients and an average of 18% drop out after enrollment. These could be the two main causes of clinical trial failure are patient recruitment and monitoring (Harrer et al., 2019). Therefore, identifying the ideal patients via precision medicine can improve the speed, efficiency, and cost-effectiveness of clinical trials overall.

AI can tackle this challenge in a variety of ways. For instance, different applications and systems based on ML and NLP can be used to mine EHRs, trial databases, social media, and other sources of data to better match patients with trials. (Lo Piano, 2020). Another example of this is Antidote, a platform that uses ML to connect patients to trials. In one trial studying Alzheimer's Disease that required 10,000 participants, Antidote was able to deliver 8,000 of those participants in less than two months. Importantly, the patients referred by Antidote were seven times more likely to complete the follow-up requirements than referrals from other sources (Antidote, 2022). It should be noted that this success was driven in great part by Antidote's partnerships—including advocacy organizations, health communities, among others—who increased traffic on Antidote's platform, demonstrating the importance of working alliances.

In terms of trial-monitoring and event reporting, AI can be deployed through wearables, which are able to transmit information in real time to researchers about participants' symptoms and events. DL can transform wearables from pure information storing and reporting devices into "cognitive sensing" devices—in other words, contextualizing and correlating this information in real time to extract meaningful insights. This is already occurring in the field of neuroscience, with wearable devices such as Embrace that are able to put together different physiological markers and interpret that an absence seizure may be happening even when an epileptic patient may not detect it (Harrer et al., 2019). Additionally, in calculating the risk of dropout from an RCT, DL and ML algorithms can take data from wearable devices and/or video monitoring to analyze what led to patient drop-out or non-adherence and can then both report these events and translate them into calculations for future patient drop-out risk (Harrer et al. 2019).

Another area in RCTs where AI can be useful is in terms of informed consent and contract drafting. AI has the ability to automate workflows and create initial drafts of standardized contracts that include vital aspects such as confidentiality, agreements, and responsibilities to expedite the process (Ford et al., 2021). Applications, such as eConsent, can be used for this purpose, presenting individualized forms to the patients, aligned with their particular sociodemographic information and along with information leaflets regarding the trials they are signing up for. In this way, this not only tackles the challenge of saving time, but also increases patient understanding and engagement.

There are important considerations regarding the role of AI in RCTs. One is the strongly regulated access to clinical data and information. In order for AI systems to analyze and create insights, they must be able to access real-world data from various sources to create cohesive profiles and insights. However, certain regulations limit AI's access to this data, and it will be vital to balance patient privacy and safety with increased access to information to improve AI. The other challenge is the explainability of AI systems (Harrer et al., 2019). Given increasing complexity, it is vital that these systems be understood and communicated in an understandable way to relevant stakeholders so that they may gain regulatory approval and mainstream acceptance.

Globally, big data, which tend to be RWD, have become an important new tool and challenge. While more data (e.g., volume, velocity, variety and veracity) can mean more insights, data first need to be processed and prepared before any meaningful analysis can take place. To prepare big data, researchers must first make sure every data point is correctly labelled, outliers have been removed or corrected, and missing cases are either removed completely or estimated properly. This process, called data cleaning, is even more salient when data is unstructured, such as that which cannot be readily stored in rows or columns in a database (i.e., clinician notes, journal articles, information from social media, etc.). Today, 80% of the world's data are unstructured, and this requires implementing additional cleaning steps that require complex algorithms. As such, data cleaning is the one of the most essential tasks in processing big, unstructured data, and can pose risks since it requires much experience and can lead to human error. For instance, statistics show that the US economy can lose up to 3 trillion dollars a year due to bad data (Redman, 2016).

To illustrate the importance and usefulness of data cleaning, let's take the example of Zillow, an online real estate database that provides listings to the general public. In order to clean its data, Zillow uses machine learning algorithms to quickly detect outliers, match data, and make a best guess of any information that might be missing from its database. For instance, if Zillow receives information about a home measuring 1,000 square feet, and initially identifies that it contains two bedrooms and 20 bathrooms, its algorithm will detect that it is highly unlikely that the bathroom information is correct. Then, the supervised algorithm can proceed to make an educated guess on what the correct number would be and quickly replace it with "2" to update the information (Gudivada et al., 2017).

Specifically, within healthcare, "dirty" or "messy" data (including missing, inconsistent or unreliable information) can disrupt HCPs access to necessary information, obstruct the path to best treatments, and delay clinical decision-making (Zand, 2020). Additionally, it becomes difficult to analyze patient trajectories and patient risk if information in a person's EHR is not clean, organized, and appropriately categorized.

Moving on to the applications in healthcare, more complex modeling such as Generative Adversarial Networks (GANs) have been used to clean and reconstruct visual data such as medical imaging. For example, a GAN-based MRI reconstruction method can clean any motion spots that may have occurred during the scan and provide a clearer and more useful image for HCPs to later analyze (Qayyum et al., 2020). According to Yi, Walia and Babym (2019), this technology has proven effective in over 150 published articles. As an added benefit, these networks may prove useful in generating standardized protocols from free-text clinical indications, improving wait times and speeding up the imaging process as a whole (Yi et al., 2019).

Another key example is Snorkel, a data programming tool that uses ML to clean data sets. In a recent study, Snorkel was used to clean data regarding organ labelling in a population-scale biomedical repository, the UK Biobank (Fries et al., 2019). Using this tool, rare aortic valve malformations were able to be classified quickly using unlabeled cardiac MRI sequences, labeling around 4,000 unlabeled cardiac MR imaging sequences, thus avoiding the need for doctors to label these manually. This effective labeling system allowed quicker identification of those at greater risk of a greater cardiac event, contributing also to faster diagnoses and patient monitoring.

Healthcare is critical worldwide, advancing now more than ever. However, it also faces increasing challenges in lieu of a changing global landscape and evolving healthcare trends. Even further, the demand for healthcare is on the rise and the human resources necessary to fill this need will not be sufficient in the near future. Considering these challenges, AI can fill a prominent gap and propel healthcare into a new era. The potential of AI in transforming healthcare is clear not across early diagnosis and prevention, clinical trials, and leveraging data for creating useful insights. This will not only benefit HCPs and the healthcare system but continue to provide greater value to patients at a lesser economic cost.

6.3 Machine and Deep Learning

As generally accepted, ML represents a sub-discipline of AI, providing specific tools and methods, where algorithms are used to describe or "learn" the relationships between input and output data, being classified in three categories: supervised (where training is based on labeled dataset), unsupervised (without a labeled dataset), and reinforcement Learning (Alsuliman, Humaidan and Sliman, 2020). Reinforcement learning is based on *punishment / reward* theory, similar to operant conditioning theory in Psychology (Skinner, 1963). The concept is simple: the system learns or adjusts based on its outcome, so multiple iterations will optimize the system specifics (parameters) or weights. The expectation is that based on the "learnt" design using training data, the system will perform well also with *alike* new data. However, training needs to be a controlled process as it could lead to overfitting. This happens when we have too many training cycles that will make the system perform very well with training data, but poor with unknown data. Overfitting is described largely in the available literature that proposes methods to avoid it (Martin Anderson, 2021). FDA also adds to the ML definition the nature of learning, either *locked* or *adaptive* (Health, 2021).

DL represents a sub-set of ML, based on neural networks, a computational model that is inspired from biologics that can have various architectures, usually layers of parallel processing nodes. The complex nature of this network gives opportunities to design simple to complex building blocks with various module designs, inputs, outputs and processing logic and matrix operations that require intensive computational power (Thompson et al., 2020). This neural network design enables applicability in multiple use cases and data domains as: image classification, object detection, structured data, question answering, named entity recognition, and machine translation. While being effective, Thompson et al. (2020) underlines the limits of DL by design. Usually, the network is initialized with random data that is computed in multiple iterations to achieve a specific goal, as minimizing a cost function or error. The model will run until a specific target is achieved and the weights (or simplistic, parameters) are established or "learnt".

A key success factor is data quality and managing the effect of the multiple sources of biases induced by data or the process of analysis. Giving the "black box" nature of the networks, the complexity and difficulty to explain the model output increases. DL architectures provide state-of-the art performance, overperforming expert systems (procedural knowledge) in multiple domains, as of 2021 benchmarks, but they can work with data sourced from multiple sources, if converted in the specific format required by algorithmic processing (Figure 6.1).

The process of using RWD to create RWE depends on some process steps, which are part of MLOps cycle (ML Operations, inspired by information technology [IT] Operations, frequently named DevOps) (Mäkinen et al., 2021).

Healthcare DL can be applied in Patient Intake; Radiology, Hematology, Neurology, Oncology, Cell Biology and Cell Therapy, Cardiology, Ophthalmology, Sports Medicine to mention just a few.

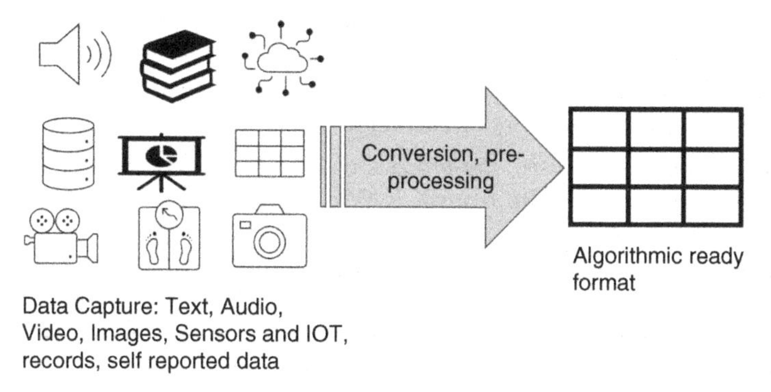

FIGURE 6.1
Real-world Data forms: formats and conversion for computing.

1. *Digitization or Data Acquisition*: available data from RWD can come in multiple formats before being suitable for ML/DL processing. The process of conversion or transformation might include the use of other ML/ DL tools. For example, RWD coming from EMR/HER, patient self-reported data, sensors, wearables (Internet of Thing) or claims may need conversion or processing using other ML powered tools. Text and scanned images might need to be captured from source systems, as well as sensory data. In retinopathy imagistic analysis, the eye fundus image needs to be captured and digitalized. In medical claims, a paper form needs to be scanned to image format and go through Optical character recognition (OCR) or Form Recognition (FR) process. Either process *might* extract text information, images, tables, and stores it in a usable format. This can be used for example to enrich the document metadata or to provide information for extracting named entities (as Person, Organization, Date, Geography using Natural Language Processing) or other relevant information so support tagging or labeling. It eliminates the need for the manual process of data extraction and provides opportunities to transform the unstructured or semi-structured image document (as a Claims Form) into a database or tabular format that can be used for analytics, similarity detection, anomaly detection, behavioral segmentation, to name a few. Text extracted paragraphs can be used for ML summarization, labels for supervised classification, text induced questions generation or training behavior-based recommendation systems. These techniques might assist the clinical act or might support other processes based on that RWD. In the case of a digital therapeutic platform, the sensor data captured regularly from wearables and other patient self-reported data can be analyzed to estimate the outcome of

the interventions and adherence for data and evidence generation of (Krishnakumar et al., 2021; Maricich et al., 2021). These examples show that additional rich features can be generated using manual labeling using human annotators or extracted using ML based methods.

2. *Data Quality Analysis, Pre-processing and Architecture Adaptation*: For example imagistic data from X-RAY or MRI will require conversion to specific format, resizing or adjustments (Lundervold and Lundervold, 2019) and the data scientists evaluates various candidate models and their architectures based on models' (to date the analysis) benchmark performance. Each data acquisition model requires its own preprocessing method. Imaging data and computer vision to be used in DL models is implemented faster if adapted to proven benchmarked CNN architectures (known as convolutional neural networks) (Khan et al., 2020). CNNs are widely discussed in literature or books. The main characteristics are that the computation is based on the principle of moving a pooling window across the image instead of using the entire image. Rather than processing large matrixes of information, the low-level features are learned based on atomic details, then being used in multiple tasks. This reduces the complexity and increases model performance. CNNs are used also in other Image Classification and Segmentation, Object Detection, Natural Language Processing, and Speech Recognition.
3. *Training:* Model training and saving is a key element of the processing as it involves the model parametric specification of architecture, iterative tuning/adjustment, model evaluation specification and actual iterations. This activity depends on the size of data, software platform, complexity of the DL network architecture and computing power. Cloud architectures allows cost efficient Cloud Computing ML processing using GPU, CPU or TPU architectures, but the usage depends on various aspects as data privacy, security (Cloud TPU, 2021; Gao and Sunyaev, 2019). For reusability and deployment in other environments a model needs to be saved. Saving the model can be done by freezing the model parameters, some architectures allowing retraining or transfer learning. Diabetic Retinopathy (DR) image classification is performed in a study, based on supervised training and labeled publicly available dataset ATOS 2019 (Khalifa et al., 2019) to support screening and diagnostic. The study considered several medium sized layers architecture as AlexNet, Res-Net18, SqueezeNet, GoogleNet, VGG16, and VGG19 against larger models, such as DenseNet or InceptionResNet and used data augmentation techniques to overcome the overfitting problem. The selected model AlexNet achieved a performance of 97.9% while its architecture provides a minimum number of layers, reducing complexity and computation effort. Thus, an exploratory analysis of the structure, the nature and quality of RWD will inform on the practical

choices of model selection. Another DR screening analysis (Wang et al., 2020) compares the results reported in literature, with observations on the characteristics of the input files considered for model training. However, the algorithm is a theoretical and mathematical proposal of an architecture, and to perform training, model load and serving it needs a platform (software framework and compatible hardware). The proposed models in published papers could have various implementations depending on the software platform and development language, if no commercial proprietary platform is selected. The most common modeling environment is open-source Python and R (Brittain et al., 2018), Python offering the advantage of being easily integrated in operational deployments using platforms, offers quick prototyping, rich integration and visualization capabilities. Transfer learning technique (ability to use learnt weights) is used to repurpose a trained model with new labeled data and requires specific tools and software methods (not all models allow it).

4. *Model Testing and Validation*: This is a critical part that needs to consider testing methodology, assess model's sensitivity, specificity, and the risk of overfitting. Due to its training specialization, supervised or unsupervised learning will perform well within the narrow space of domain knowledge (for example X-Ray and MRI classifiers should be deployed on separate models) and that adds complexity from a ML Ops perspective, requiring tools, infrastructure and processes in place. Cross-validations may also be conducted.
5. *Model Loading and Serving:* This is a critical capability to allow model storage and reload, versioning and reuse, due to its intensive computational nature. A saved model is a collection of files stored on the drive in a specific format. If a complex CNN architecture might take days and expensive infrastructure to train, the model should be able to be saved and reload. Serving from a saved model should be very fast and support generating outputs. In practice, multiple steps of data preparation, processing of training data will apply in operational platforms to *new* data like cleaning, transformation, so the two processes are linked and should be synced.
6. *Model Lifecycle*: this is part of the AI Governance, versioning control and established process, decision makers and RACI matrixes. This should follow principles in Software Development Lifecycle and ITIL methodologies part of IT Governance (Iden and Eikebrokk, 2014) including the specifics of the ML/ DL practice.

The topic of ML/DL is very broad, so the next paragraph will mention some of the frameworks used in healthcare with examples:

- Pytorch (Paszke et al., 2019.): provides a versatile, Python library, optimized for tensors processing (tensor represent a matrix) and is used to design and train DL neural networks and can be used for computer vision and natural language processing, a versatile and efficient library. For model serving and production, it depends on other frameworks. A proposed CNNs architecture, using ResNet-50 model trained on Mosmed-1110 dataset was used to classify Covid 19 cases using 3D CT Scans (Serte and Demirel, 2021). The paper provides detail on Pytorch model implementation, training time and hardware platform. AllenNLP (allenai/allennlp-models, 2021) is built on top of Pytorch and provides state of the art tasks implementation and pretrained models for classification, Coreference resolution (finding all of the expressions in a text that refer to common entities), Language Modelling, Named Entity Recognition.
- SpaCy (spaCy 101: Everything you need to know spaCy. Usage Documentation, 2021) and ScispaCy (Neumann et al., 2019). Spacy is a full featured, production ready library that offers many methods for NLP, including pipelines, visualization, annotation methods as well the ability to train custom models. Spacy is used to extract features from text and supports building specialized NLP libraries on top of it, as ScispaCy (AllenAI, trained on biomedical literature, offering ready to use, pretrained models). These greatly accelerate the effort of tagging documents with disease related information, chemical or medical abbreviation, for example. This augmentation can support other downstream classification or segmentation tasks. A study evaluating the improvement of reproducibility of clinical trials using features extracted with seven NLP tools (Digan et al., 2021) from articles published in PubMed and Web of Science, found that scispaCy (as a NLP toolkit trained on the BIONLP13CG biomedical corpora) is able to provide partial functionality comparing to other workflow based frameworks, matching 17 out of 40 reproducibility features. Another study used scispaCy to process data to evaluate the extraction of named entities on a limited corpus (Tarcar et al., 2020).
- Tensorflow (Google) is another state-of-the art framework, and Keras were used in application as Skin Cancer images Classifications using a CNN architecture trained using the HAM10000 training dataset (Benbrahim, Hachimi and Amine, 2020). Keras (Chollet and others, 2018) was used on top of Tensorflow as a high level library that simplifies the modeling and training, to classify seven types of skin cancer. Tensorflow is used in imagistic as breast cancer classification (Chang and Chung, 2020; Adeshina et al., 2018), lung cancer classification (Cengil and Cinar, 2018). Tensorflow also provides a robust operationalization or mobile/web browser deployments for client-side serving.

- NLP-oriented models and their python implementations, that allows rapid experimentation: T5 (Raffel et al., 2020), known as text to text transformer uses pretrained models (Xue et al., 2021; T5: Text-To-Text Transfer Transformer, 2021) to quickly solve tasks such as machine translation, question answering from paragraph, document summarization, classification using transfer learning using the mechanism of attention. T5 is partially inspired by Unified Language Model (Howard and Ruder, 2018), ULMFit being implementation in python as an open-source library, FastAI (Howard and Gugger, 2020). This approach comes from computer vision transfer learning but can use text (NLP), images or tabular data. A novel approach of word vector representation was word2vec (Mikolov et al., 2013), proposing an efficient way to represent words into a vector space and allow similarity calculations based on method as cosine similarity. In short, based on a corpus trained, we are able to detect proximity in the vector space or visualize in 2D or 3D, a PCA reduced vector space. This can suggest association between molecules, diseases or similarity and is a form of unsupervised learning using shallow neural networks. A popular python package that allows word2vec software implementation is Gensim (Řehůřek and Sojka, 2010).
- Generative Adversarial Network (GAN), added a new opportunity proposing adversarial nets (Goodfellow et al., 2014) by opposing similar models (e.g., Generative and Discriminative) in a two agents game environment.
- OpenAI and its famous GPT3 language model (Wilson and Daugherty, 2020) is a generative model, that used a large amount of training data and is not yet ready to replace a human conversational agent. A paper (Korngiebel and Mooney, 2021) evaluated the healthcare opportunities opened by this massive model, trained on 175 Bn parameters, found biases and errors, related to gender, ethnicity or race, generated from the training corpuses, suggesting that even if it performs well on benchmark corpuses, it does not represent Artificial General Intelligence and cannot be a substitute for Human Intelligence, despite performing well on free-form conversations. The paper also suggests potential healthcare use cases, such as automation, documentation, processing of EHR, under Human supervision and potentially as chatbot agents.

The capabilities offered by these libraries provide new opportunities but also challenges. Thus, what are the advances occurring in ML/DL in conjunction with RWD and challenges that would need to be overcome to enhance the effectiveness of the usage of ML/DL? We see that data types and value-added use cases are influencing the adoption of AI, DL and ML in healthcare. For example, specialized and repeatable tasks, such as image classification or imagistic tagging annotation could benefit DL or ML technologies, while other tasks, such as natural language has multiple challenges due to its semi-structure nature. However, these tools can augment or suggest a new direction to support the generation of RWE.

The biggest challenges in RWD remain data and process related biases. Some of them are part of the research methodology in other disciplines, where qualitative or quantitative research methods are used. The National Institute of Standards and Technology (NIST, 2021) has drafted a proposal for identifying and managing bias in AI. Here we describe a few potential biases due to the following reasons.

- Data and data acquisition (Saunders, Lewis and Thornhill, 2009)
  - Historical bias
  - Representation bias (definition and sample from a population)
  - Population bias (dataset is not representative to population statistics)
  - Sampling bias (non-random sampling)
  - Data collection and measurement error
  - Disparate systems with different ontologies and taxonomies.
- Algorithm induced (Mehrabi et al., 2019)
  - Evaluation bias (during model validation)
  - Popularity bias (news, search results, behavioral associations)
  - Omitted variable bias
  - Correlated variables bias (inter-item similarity)
  - Chained models and propagation of error
- Interpretation induced
  - Measurement bias (how choose and measure a particular feature)
  - Aggregation bias (how we generalize based on subgroup)
  - Behavioral bias (e.g., emoji usage in social media)
  - Cause-Effect bias (e.g., correlation versus causation; The Stork-and-Baby Trap, 2021)

Giving the nature of "real-life" RWD collection within a process, it is probable that data reflects partially the overall target universe related to the study scope. The main factors contributing to the bias (Panch, Mattie and Atun, 2019) comes from:

1. Lack of fairness (subpopulation representations, due to the nature of process collecting RWD or BigData)

2. Lack of contextual specificity (a general AI should consider rich diversity, while population characteristics are localized)
3. Black box nature of DL models (or explain-ability of the models)

To overcome the risk of bias, data scientists and researchers need to look for solutions to mitigate these effects. On the other hand, AI or DL is not a mean end. There are cases when different solutions or approaches are more valuable. This shouldn't hinder the DL or ML opportunity in healthcare, but suggests the need for regulation and guidance, formats harmonization that might take long or be impractical. These changes are real and here to stay. While hypertext transfer protocol (HTTP)standardize the way that Internet works, despite the connectivity, the format of the data itself still generates a lot of challenges in performing analysis on crawled data. Organizations developing practices and having solid data foundation in place are advantaged, as Data Science is a heavily data intensive process requiring Data Governance. Data privacy and ethical considerations are critical for the value for the patient delivered by healthcare using RWD in different jurisdictions.

6.4 Personal Devices Augmenting User Experience

Before describing the value provided by personal devices is recommended to provide the current definition as devices for patient or healthcare, that are "portable, consumer-focused technologies that assist with remote monitoring." "Examples of these devices include thermometers, pulse oximeters, blood pressure cuffs, pedometers, weight scales, fitness equipment, medication tracking, and glucose meters." (Eramo, 2010) or "Sensors, wearable or not, are devices with constrained resources, specially related to energy supply and processing power" that called Personal Health Devices (PHDs) (Santos, Perkusich and Almeida, 2014) and are commonly associated with Internet of Things (IOT) or Internet of Medical Things (IOMT) and their connectivity, associated frequently to mobile apps/ smart devices.

The proposed Healthcare 4.0 (Aceto, Persico and Pescapé, 2020) framework identifies in a systematic review a series of applications around internet of things (IoT), internet of medical things (IoMT), big data and cloud computing around rehabilitation, assisted living, telehealth and disease monitoring, cloud health information systems, personalized healthcare, smart pharmaceuticals and medication intake monitoring, self-managed wellness and monitoring pathological and physiological signals, just to name a few, based on "anywhere-anytime connectivity." This view is patient-centric, while such devices can be used to also augment HCP experience for learning and exchanging information with patients. However, the data stored using a personal device might pose security compliance and risks as well privacy concerns (Bromwich and Bromwich, 2016) in case that patient is sharing private information.

Mobile apps via mobile health (mHealth) can be used as standalone or can use connected devices as wearables to facilitate communication between mobile app and service provider to synchronize or retrieve data. Mobile phones have a series of sensors that can help capturing and generating RWD that can be stored and analyzed centrally, on edge, at mobile device level. Many ML trained models implemented in mobile frameworks can benefit from additional privacy by computing the outcome of the model without concerns of sending the data externally. TensorFlow Lite is an example of such a framework that works on smartphones (TensorFlow Lite | ML for Mobile and Edge Devices, 2021). This approach keeps all data locally stored, and the service provider cannot benefit of data collection. The data coming from devices can be in detecting various physical activities as pedestrian behavior and risk of walking using smartphone (Kareem et al., 2021) applying a ML algorithm on data generated by smartphone's gyroscope with accuracy over 90% or activity classification by use of accelerometer or fall detection using mobile's accelerometer and gyroscopic data using a cloud ML models served in Real Time (Mrozek, Koczur and Małysiak-Mrozek, 2020). Alternative design options exist if the apps deploy or downloads the ML model in a ML mobile app for local serving. The amount of data is constantly fed in a prediction model that can trigger a series of interventions as needed or personalized interaction. That can be useful to mitigate the risk of post-surgery fall or other types of falls in monitored patients, in home or facility settings. Applications are multiple and can generate value for both patients and providers (healthcare, insurers, care takers). However, the accuracy of the data is not suitable for any critical use case. For example, in Parkinson's disease, detection of tremor, bradykinesia, gait impairment, and motor complications, such as dyskinesia are not easily done by smartphone in a home-setting (Espay et al., 2016). The same study also underlines the lack of motivation and abandonment rate of mobile apps.

Adoption or abandonment is linked to the perceptual motivational constructs from TAM (Davis, 1989) that explain the perceived usefulness and ease of use as common factors influencing behavioral intention to use. Thus, the quality of content, interaction and user experience is a factor that influences application adoption rate. Potentially, a gamified experience might improve adherence even if based on extrinsic motivators or rewards, such as badges, levels, and awards that are not constant in time compared to extrinsic motivation. The role of intrinsic motivation against extrinsic and theory effect on behavior was discussed by Deci and Ryan (2000) in

SDT, Self-determination theory proposed in 1985, as well as distinction between internal and external motives. The psychological effect of application adoption in a health-related setup should have a broader coverage. A study focused on understanding the adherence of anti-depressant medication compared SDT with other two theories, self-regulation model and health belief model, and finds SDT combined with motivational interviewing (Miller and Rollnick, 2012) to improve motivation for adherence and increase autonomy. Motivational Interviewing is not a theory but a direct, non-confrontational clinical communication strategy that elicits with intrinsic motivation (Hamrin, Sinclair and Gardner, 2017).

Pose analytics and real-time high-frequency data can also be generated by using computer vision on edge devices by generating stream of data with coordinates related to pose on image or video feed. Additional downstream ML models can be used to classify and predict the class of behavior or describe a specific behavior. TensorFlow Lite (Pose estimation | TensorFlow Lite, 2021) released a pretrained model that can be used for and detects body joints and provide graphical representation for segments.

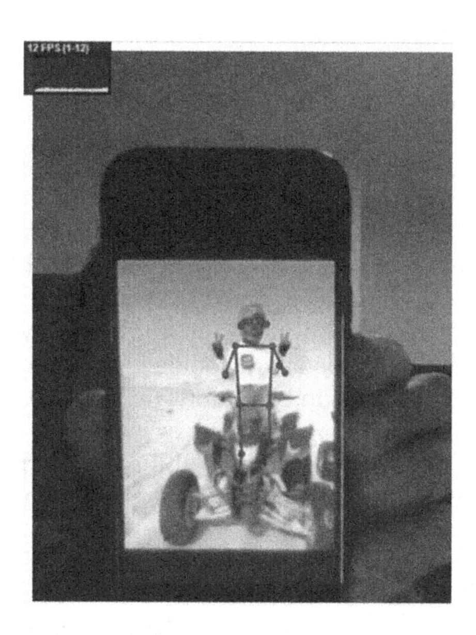

FIGURE 6.2
Posenet 2.0 model serving, based on MobileNet v1. Image captured by author's experiment using browser-based real time pose detection on laptop camera stream from smartphone displaying an image of a quad rider wearing helmet. The model is able to detect some joints while failing to detect the vehicle details in a non-optimal data capture context.

The quality of the joint and movement identification may not be acceptable at image level but if used in video analytics can detect and use classification algorithms for movement detection, fall detection, static position detection (Figure 6.2). By edge serving the captured by Posenet 2.0 remains local, while application can trigger interventions based on specific protocols, based on predicted score, and joints position over a specific period. Other activities related to fitness, wellness, rehabilitations can be modeled and implemented, while the RWD generation is delegated to Posenet or similar models. Other applications can use Augmented or Virtual Reality for linking physical behavior detection with a set of system responses.

Medication use, intake, fill and time on medication are key behaviors and measures for adherence across HCPs and healthcare ecosystems, especially MCDs (Singh, Bhatnagar and Moond, 2017). Patients with mental illness as bipolar disorder can receive intentions as psychoeducation and cognitive behavioral therapies (CBTs) delivered by smart device. Adherence can be improved by alerts and survey taking. Other apps targeted schizophrenia patients medicine intake monitoring using simple interventions as alerts or scheduler functionality while also providing support for physician–patient conversation (Bianco et al., 2021). Other devices that can be used are smart pill dispensers (Aldeer, Javanmard and Martin, 2018) that can improve adherence by direct measurement along with other methods as wearable, ingestible bio-sensors, RFID or NFC communication devices and computer vision.

Beside sensors, smartphones have incorporated increasingly high-quality cameras that can assist telemedicine and capturing images. For example, skin cancer detection apps might not have the expected accuracy while two apps have approval as software medical devices by European regulators but only one found reliable in a systematic review (Freeman et al., 2020), while also the healthcare professionals express concerns on available apps that are not regulated in App stores (Wise 2018). The FDA names this app MMAs (Health, 2020). While the FDA has not approve any application yet, due to increased concerns it is expected to happen and Google recently announced its interest in applying AI for detecting skin conditions (MD, 2021). The announcement clearly stated that it is not a diagnosis tool or a software medical device (Bui 2021), but for targeting to improve HCPs' ability to interpret skin conditions. This strategy was to continue developing the product, while describing the tool as SMD.

Diabetic condition management can benefit from mobile apps and devices (Fleming et al., 2020) and comorbidities. Mobile apps focused on diet and exercise were found to be effective and have a positive effect on short term (less than 12 months) in glycemic control while contradictory results were found for long term (Represas-Carrera, Martínez-Ques and Clavería, 2021) based on a systematic review.

HCPs can benefit through use of mobile devices if Virtual Reality (VR) or Augmented Reality (AR) is used in patient education, procedure education giving the processing power of the devices, as well as the interactivity that these types of apps are providing with a relative low cost (Moro et al., 2017).

A study (Menni et al., 2020) used the mobile app to collect self-reported data for COVID19 symptoms for condition prediction using Supervised ML proposing a regression model for model explainability. It involved approximatively 2.6. million participants in the UK and US in 2020, for less than a month, an impressive number in a short period of time.

The usage of devices also raises concerns that need to be addressed. Security and data privacy, the impact of time-zone and travel over reminders, software updates and risk of exposing private or sensitive data. Due to the nature of edge device, the data encryption is a concern (IoT Security Issues: Top 10 Challenges, 2020; Karale, 2021) and the IT industry is expected to address this by guidance on security standards and their adoption.

6.5 Process to Identify a Potential Technology Solution

Regardless of the technology used, the interest in applicability of ML or AI in the field of healthcare is constantly increasing. Plotting the numbers of

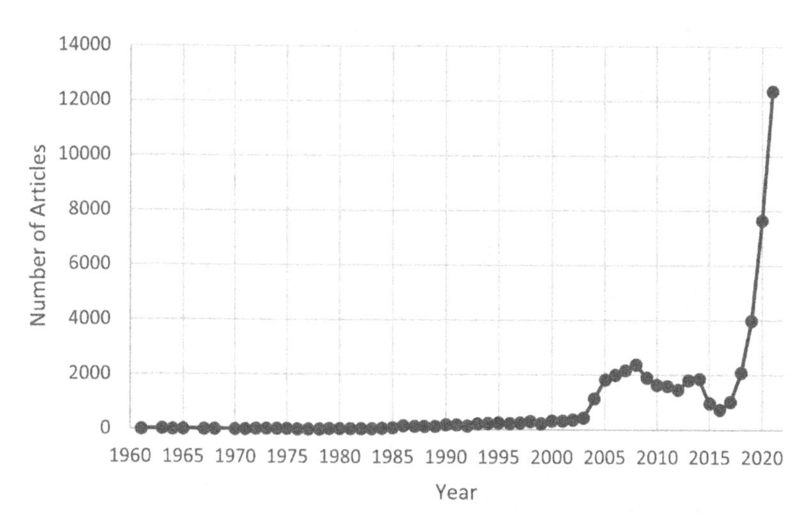

FIGURE 6.3
Source PubMed, author exploratory analysis.

literature reviews available in PubMed using the search term "artificial intelligence", shows an increasing high interest since 2017, with a record number 2,080 "Review" category papers published in 2020 (Figure 6.3).

However, the adoption of advanced analytics within the organization depends on multiple factors, such as People, Process, Technology, and Governance. Applications of Artificial Intelligence in Healthcare, in a general acceptance, improve processes such as detection, diagnosis, treatment, and the prediction of the outcome (Kumar, Gadag and Nayak, 2021). Giving the complexity or real world data (RWD), diversity of sources, there are both challenges and opportunities from the *volume* (also mentioned as BigData), *velocity* and *variety* (What is big data? More than volume, velocity and variety 2017), adding later the data quality aspect, called *veracity*.

In data analytics, the processes and methods of preparation, cleansing and transformation are critical for accuracy or quality of models. The digital records under RWD (e.g., claims, EHR, EMR, social media or patient generated data) are heavily affected by sampling error or bias that affects the generation of Real-world Evidence by causal inference (Crown, 2019). Using traditional RCT methods, these biases are minimized and accepted practice, while in RWD they reflect real patient behavior and clinical response but could pose challenges when generalizing the study's findings. This bias is not new and is commonly treated in multiple discipline research methods as social sciences research methodologies or marketing research (Saunders, Lewis and Thornhill, 2009). A suggestive case of non-representative sampling for US presidential pre-election pools was recorded in 1936 (Wang et al., 2015), over a sample of 2 million responses, a huge number for that time, collected by a popular magazine, *Literary Digest*. The bias led to incorrect prediction of the victory, due to the selection criteria used (telephone, auto or subscribers), the results being valid for the sample, but not being able to generalize to the entire US population.

Natually, RWD poses some challenges in the process of identifying technical solutions that are not prevalent for processes with more structured data or standardized data sources. The properties of "BigData" sources might delay the adoption of technology while paying the opportunity cost of RWD value existing within enterprises.

Here, we focus on technology and associated process for using the technology although the capability and skillset of data science echo systems are also critical. The process of proposing a technology solution needs to be focused on problem solving or uncovering the unmet needs of the organization based on internal or external data. As mentioned before, data represents and electronic representation of a physical phenomenon or fact that was converted into data format, using a set of conventions, tools, and sensors. Simply put, beside the formal meaning or interpretation of an image, text, sound, signals, digital or analog sensors (generally named IOT, Internet of Things) or waves, in electronic systems data is represented in most cases in a binary format, being able to be processed numerically in various formats (numbers, vectors). Other architectures are non-binary, as quantum computing (Watson et al., 2018; Leprince-Ringuet, 2021). Thus, the process of data capture, ingestion, transformation, and harmonization is a critical part of the process. Traditionally BigData platforms don't directly handle the data capture and digitization, but integrates, consumes, and aggregates the data in common formats.

Data format and integration is a key concern of the large scale or dimension of RWD for its usability due to the lack of standardization, requiring adopting companies to invest in tools and processes, that are based on so called BigData Reference Architectures (Sultanow et al., 2018; [Reference Architecture] ACR-AI Lab Hospital Reference Architecture Framework, 2021; Rodriguez, 2020; Maggsl, 2021). Over time, big technology players provided technology-focused frameworks to guide companies on taking the right choices for architecture and solution design, shifting from big data to AI architectures. Due to the heavy computation involved in deep learning, transfer learning on massive amounts of data, specialized hardware was used as Graphical Cards GPU – dedicated computing unit optimized for matrix operations (Deep Learning, 2015) or TPU, proprietary hardware from Google, optimized for Tensorflow, an end to end open-source platform for ML (Cloud TPU, 2021). There is also a tendency to separate the reference architecture between conceptual building blocks, functional building blocks or technology building-blocks. For example, vendors will provide guidance in selecting the building blocks for workload virtualization, data pipelines for extraction, transformation and load, serverless computing to build a modular cloud or hybrid solution design (Sdgilley, 2021), but there is a significant effort in integrating into existing Healthcare Information systems. Cloud adoption and its influencing factors in Healthcare depends on the context and should be tailored to the AI vision aligned with the company's data strategy (Gao and Sunyaev, 2019), a study based the analysis across 67 relevant articles from a sample of 2185. With the accelerated technological advancement, a design-oriented methodology might not be actual in one year, while architectural principles of solution design are valid regardless of technology building blocks. One powerful Enterprise Architecture method is available for organization and strong guidance for practitioners is made available by The Open Group (The TOGAF® Standard, Version 9.2, 2021).

The process of selecting a technology should start with the *business research questions* or unmet healthcare needs—*known or unknown*. Statistical methods in the exploratory data analysis applied to big data are still relevant but require specific tools (Scott, 2018), as this will generate new questions or assess the data quality for its variables, allowing researchers to propose the addition or exclusion of categorical variables or to propose common factor analysis, based on domain knowledge. Various methods, such as bias, outlier detection, multiple collinearity, and visualization can be used to understand the structure and quality of the data. The decision of data integration, harmonization in common formats should follow the research question needs. Beside the data analysis, in some cases qualitative research methods can be used to understand the specific of the collected datasets and uncover unmet needs. Real-world Data usage might raise ethical and privacy concerns and concerns on the initial nature of data collection (Lipworth, 2019).

For general acceptance, the ML algorithms are used to validate hypothesis or generate hypothesis and poses significant challenges due to its complexity (Shaw et al., 2019; Jackson and Hu, 2019). From a platform perspective, the operationalization phase is different than exploration and requires a different set of capabilities to integrate an ML model in an application or production environment. That requires adoption of specific hardware and software components, part of the solution architecture, regardless of if provided as a cloud computing environment or a dedicated, on-premises computing farm. Architectural frameworks could be conceptual or more technology oriented, specific to vendors, providing guidance in integrating various technological building blocks (or components) that serves dedicated roles in information processing (integration, transformation, data catalog, modeling). Thus, it is not advisable for a large RWD project to start with a fully functional technical architecture without going to the exploratory phase, also known as minimum viable product (MVP; Ries, 2011), a term that describes the need to explore the "fit for purpose" of a solution, with incremental adjustments rather than a big deployment. This allows stakeholders to make the right cost-effective decisions, while dealing with the uncertainty of a final product. Multiple vendors shift from a fully integrated technology stack approach to a loosely coupled approach, due to the nature of cloud computing that enables gradual adoption of technology capabilities (Minevich, 2021), calling it either "pragmatic" based on building blocks or maturity model. The AI Enterprise Maturity Model also represents a tool to measure the readiness and status of the people, process, technology and governance view, multiple frameworks being available. This assessment is important, because AI adoption might be successful in isolated or departmental experiments, but organization lacks the opportunity in using its potential and scale.

Technology may not always be adopted in a timely fashion, despite the value provided even if available, and AI is no different. Technology Acceptance Model (Davis, 1989), derived from theory of planned behavior (TPB; Ajzen, 1991), was used to explain the success or failure of multiple technology adoption studies, based on motivational states as perceived usefulness and perceived ease of use that effects the Behavioral Intention to be used. TAM was developed later in other variants and adapted to specific areas of research as learning, social media, internet and mobile application (Tamilmani et al., 2021). In practice, that suggests that technology alone cannot provide the value without proper methodologies. Some companies provide guidance in a selection of AI platforms, taking into account multiple factors as ease of use, scalability or integration, as well as considering ethical considerations (Char, Shah and Magnus, 2018; Taulli, 2021b).

Choosing the right methodology to uncover the customer insights and unmet needs, followed by the process of technology selection should follow qualitative research methods followed by quantitative of data insights driven methods. While data generated is growing every year due to the technology advancements and adoption, AI or ML models are based on mathematical computations and the goal to achieve a specific target, as minimizing a specific set of parameters (as error) or finding the best model to achieve a target. There are software packages or platforms that aim to identify the best candidate algorithm from a pool of known techniques using various data sources, such as EHR or claims data, recognizing that each unique data structure poses a different challenge, requiring also automated feature engineering (Waring, Lindvall and Umeton, 2020), but still requires a significant effort in data quality assessment, feature validation and model interpretation. Sometimes, even if performing well with high sensitivity in clinical studies, the AI models can show weak results as noted by studying the efficacy of AI driven DR diagnosis, a complication of diabetes melius, of seven AI solutions (Lee et al., 2021).

Selecting between commercial platforms, open-source or custom-build is a matter of choice, depending on the existing organizational capabilities. The availability of open-source software such as Python or R software languages, the availability of public or commercial datasets and the choice of cost-efficient "pay as you go" cloud-computing platforms specializing in AI, ML and DL created a unique opportunity to break the entry barrier of expensive infrastructure and software licensing. Python also became the preferred "full stack engineering" platform, that allows not only training the ML models, but also serving as micro-services (Raschka, Patterson and Nolet, 2020). However, the serving and modeling environment is only a layer of the Reference architecture that includes the need to handle massive amounts of RWD, which has been generated or aggregated. Recognizing the rich capabilities of Python and R, many AI platform providers allow custom extensions in Python and R, to leverage the existing packages. Those are "scripting" languages and avoid vendor lock-in with proprietary methods, as in the case of compiled binary programs. According to Statista, in April 2019, US, the most required skill in data science programming is Python with a score of 76.13% followed by R, with 57.9% (Most wanted data science skills US, 2019; 2021).

Operationalizing a model or model serving requires additional organizational capabilities and investment to be able to integrate an ML model and expose it as a micro-service (A Quick Primer on Microservices – DZone Integration, 2021; SOA vs. Microservices: What's the Difference?, 2021), application or integrate it as a AI Platform service that provides an application specific functionality. A model is expected to consume new data and provide

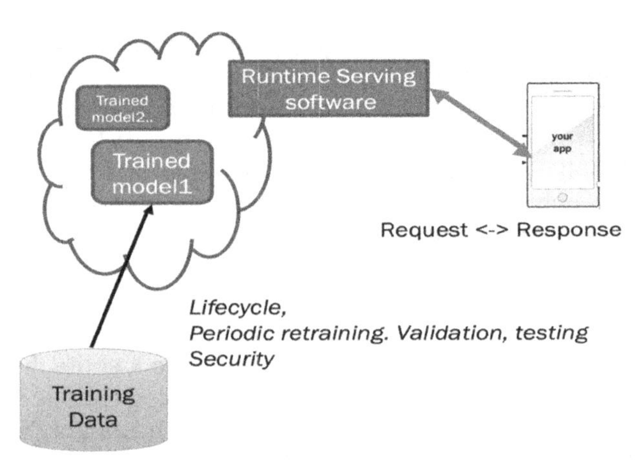

FIGURE 6.4
Conceptual simplified representation of model training and serving in real-time.

the expected output in a needed format. A trained model can be used offline or in near-real time to extract and enhance a specific dataset while others will need to be available in real-time (Figure 6.4).

The approach of having an abstract layer for the application provides the flexibility to integrate AI in a micro-service-oriented architecture, reduces the dependencies of the application from the ML complexity and also allows AI services to integrate legacy or custom applications. This allows organizations to leverage existing practice in building or integrating software applications while providing the necessary flexibility required by ML algorithms. Modern architectures avoid monolith applications and use communication endpoints between micro-services as REST API (What is a REST API?, 2021) services to communicate in a loosely coupled solution design. This mimics the web communication protocol, simplifying the connectivity between application modules, providing an easy and standard integration model. Not all deployments need to be operationalized as fully integrated models. To enable data science and statistical work as solid data foundation enablers, as data provisioning and sandboxing, data catalog, critical capabilities of Data Governance are needed (Janssen et al., 2020). This chapter discusses the details of applying Data Governance for AI in detail and provides an overview to help practitioners understand their organizational gaps.

Several examples of real-time platforms FDA approved might be relevant, as they were implemented as real-time technology solutions.

1. An AI-driven service received FDA's permit (Commissioner, 2020) as the first AI diagnostic system in 2018 based on a clinical study of retinal images obtained from 874 patients to detect more than mild positive

conditions. The solution (IDx-DR, 2021) uses a specialized fundus camera to capture two images per eye followed by AI service processing and diagnosis, providing immediate results. The use of the camera to generate fundus images, to feed a predictive model demonstrates how a trained model can be used in an end-to-end AI application. The model training used a publicly available dataset of labeled images, Messidor-2 (Decencière et al., 2014; Abramoff et al., 2016).

2. Another example of the use of Digital Therapeutics is for treating Chronic Insomnia, by providing a web based CBT-I (Cognitive Behavioral Therapy for Insomnia, a psychological intervention) platform showing robust clinical efficacy, providing salience stimulus using mobile capabilities or sleep diary, being a cost-effective treatment (Morin, 2020). This combines various technologies to deliver a specific clinical outcome.

Remarks

The selection of a health technology solution should be paired with the AI and Data Governance process (Taulli, 2021a) and data readiness. Even with incremental adoption, the AI's maturity level of the organization will provide a robust foundation for scaling, that takes into account not only technical, but also security, ethical and social implications (Gasser and Almeida, 2017).

The testing methodology should follow the accepted software industry practices and methodologies, specific to the ML orAI frameworks, with tailored considerations related to model product's lifecycle, continuous data quality assessment and bias monitoring, in both training and production environments.

Currently, the increasing use of AI or ML models to understand data, generate new insights or inferences provides a new opportunity. Thiswas not possible without the technology proliferation, reduction of processing costs, democratization of datasets, rich choice of opensource libraries and pre-trained models. However, moving from a research or prototype to operational AI or ML to deployment requires significant changes in the IT environments, but can provide new capabilities. The pragmatic approach of data-based experiments or exploratory research, evaluation of current biases and mitigation of its effects can help in improving results. The goal should be answering the business questions on top of available evidence from the data and not AI or ML, those being just a tool for better outcomes. Sometimes the available data is not ready for building an ML model aimed to automate a specific process as it assumes repetitive sequences of data-in/data-out flows with expected (accepted) confidence levels but the techniques can be used to explain the current gaps in the data or inform the needs of the data quality.

Last, but not the least, an AI-focused approaches can systematically drive more efficiencies and manage the AI governance process, e.g., via automation, compared to a distributed or isolated practice (Davenport and Dasgupta 2021), supporting creation of the AI vision, business driven use cases, target architecture, collaboration, development of skills and practice, manage internal innovation.

Disclaimer

Joseph P. Cook, Gabriel Jipa, and Lobna A. Salem are employees of Viatris, merged between Upjohn, a Division of Pfizer, and Mylan. Claudia Zavata is a former contractor of Upjohn, a Division of Pfizer, and Viatris. The views expressed are the authors' own and do not necessarily represent those of their employer or employers. The authors appreciate the editorial support from Arghya Bhattacharya and Aswin Kumar A of Viatris.

References

Abramoff, M.D., Lou, Y., Erginay, A., Clarida, W., Amelon, R., Folk, J.C. and Niemeijer, M. Improved Automated Detection of Diabetic Retinopathy on a Publicly Available Dataset Through Integration of Deep Learning. Investigative Ophthalmology & Visual Science, 2016; 57(13): 5200–5206. https://doi.org/10.1167/iovs.16-19964 KHZ (Accessed on March 30, 2022).

Aceto, G., Persico, V. and Pescapé, A. Industry 4.0 and Health: Internet of Things, Big Data, and Cloud Computing for Healthcare 4.0. Journal of Industrial Information Integration, 2020; 18: 100–129. https://doi.org/10.1016/j.jii.2020.100129 KHZ (Accessed on March 30, 2022).

Adeshina, S.A., Adedigba, A.P., Adeniyi, A.A. and Aibinu, A.M. 2018. Breast Cancer Histopathology Image Classification with Deep Convolutional Neural Networks. In: 2018 14th International Conference on Electronics Computer and Computation (icecco). [online] New York: Ieee. www.webofscience.com/wos/woscc/full-record/WOS:000462760400011 Industry 4.0 and Health: Internet of Things, Big Data, and Cloud Computing for Healthcare 4.0 (Accessed on March 30, 2022).

Ajzen, I. The theory of planned behavior. Organizational Behavior and Human Decision Processes, 1991; 50(2): 179–211. https://doi.org/10.1016/0749-5978(91)90020-T Industry 4.0 and Health: Internet of Things, Big Data, and Cloud Computing for Healthcare 4.0 (Accessed March 30, 2022).

Aldeer, M., Javanmard, M. and Martin, R.P. A Review of Medication Adherence Monitoring Technologies. Applied System Innovation, 2018; 1(2): 14. https://doi.org/10.3390/asi1020014 (Accessed on March 30, 2022).
Alsuliman, T., Humaidan, D. and Sliman, L. Machine learning and artificial intelligence in the service of medicine: Necessity or potentiality? Current Research in Translational Medicine, 2020; 68(4): 245–251. https://doi.org/10.1016/j.retram.2020.01.002 (Accessed on March 30, 2022).
American College of Obstetricians and Gynecologists, press release June 26, 2020. www.acog.org/news/news-articles/2020/06/acog-wins-private-insurers-extending-covid-19-telehealth-policies. See also KFF, www.kff.org/womens-health-policy/issue-brief/opportunities-and-barriers-for-telemedicine-in-the-u-s-during-the-covid-19-emergency-and-beyond/ (Accessed on March 30, 2022).
American Hospital Association. Assessing AI's Potential for Care Delivery. 2020. www.aha.org/aha-center-health-innovation-market-scan/2019-12-03-assessing-ais-potential-care-delivery (Accessed on March 30, 2022).
Antidote. Where patients meet research.2022. www.antidote.me (Accessed on March 30, 2022).
Bailey, M. As virtual doctor visits take off, debate over who should pay heats up, STAT 2016. www.statnews.com/2016/03/22/telemedicine-reimbursement/ (Accessed on March 30, 2022).
Bali S. Barriers to development of telemedicine in developing countries. In: Heston TF (ed)Telehealth. 2018; IntechOpen, London, UK, 10.5772/intechopen.81723 (Accessed March 30, 2022).
Benbrahim, H., Hachimi, H. and Amine, A. Deep Convolutional Neural Network with Tensorflow and Keras to Classify Skin Cancer Images. Scalable Computing-Practice and Experience, 2020; 21(3): 379–389. https://doi.org/10.12694/scpe.v21i3.1725 (Accessed on March 30, 2022).
Benke K, Benke G. Artificial Intelligence and Big Data in Public Health. Int J Environ Res Public Health. 2018 Dec 10;15(12):2796.
Bianco, C.L., Myers, A.L., Smagula, S. and Fortuna, K.L. Can Smartphone Apps Assist People with Serious Mental Illness in Taking Medications as Prescribed? Sleep Medicine Clinics, 2021; 16(1): 213–222. https://doi.org/10.1016/j.jsmc.2020.10.010 (Accessed on March 30, 2022).
Booz Allen Hamilton. Intelligence. 2022. www.boozallen.com/markets/intelligence.html (Accessed on March 30, 2022).
Brittain, J., Cendon, M., Nizzi, J. and Pleis, J. Data Scientist's Analysis Toolbox: Comparison of Python, R, and SAS Performance. 2018; 1(2): 20.
Bui P. Using AI to help find answers to common skin conditions. Google. 2021. https://blog.google/technology/health/ai-dermatology-preview-io-2021/ https://blog.google/technology/health/ai-dermatology-preview-io-2021 (Accessed on March 30, 2022).
Bromwich, M. and Bromwich, R. Privacy risks when using mobile devices in health care. CMAJ: Canadian Medical Association Journal, 2016; 188(12): 855–856. https://doi.org/10.1503/cmaj.160026 (Accessed on March 30, 2022).
Cengil, E. and Cinar, A. A Deep Learning Based Approach to Lung Cancer Identification. In: 2018 International Conference on Artificial Intelligence and Data Processing (idap). 2018; New York: Ieee. www.webofscience.com/wos/woscc/full-record/WOS:000458717400004 (Accessed on March 30, 2022).

Chang, Y.-H. and Chung, C.-Y. Classification of Breast Cancer Malignancy Using Machine Learning Mechanisms in TensorFlow and Keras. In: K.P. Lin, R. Magjarevic and P. DeCarvalho, eds. Future Trends in Biomedical and Health Informatics and Cybersecurity in Medical Devices, Icbhi 2019. 2020; Cham: Springer International Publishing Ag: 42–49. https://doi.org/10.1007/978-3-030-30636-6_6 (Accessed on March 30, 2022).

Char, D.S., Shah, N.H. and Magnus, D. Implementing Machine Learning in Health Care — Addressing Ethical Challenges. The New England Journal of Medicine, 2018; 378(11): 981–983. https://doi.org/10.1056/NEJMp1714229 (Accessed on March 30, 2022).

Chen L, Carlton Jones AL, Mair G, Patel R, Gontsarova A, Ganesalingam J, Math N, Dawson A, Aweid B, Cohen D, Mehta A, Wardlaw J, Rueckert D, Bentley P; IST-3 Collaborative Group. Rapid Automated Quantification of Cerebral Leukoaraiosis on CT Images: A Multicenter Validation Study. Radiology. 2018 Aug;288(2):573–581..

Chollet, F. and others. Keras: The Python Deep Learning library. Astrophysics Source Code Library, 2018; p.ascl:1806.022. Available at: https://ui.adsabs.harvard.edu/abs/2018ascl.soft06022C (Accessed on March 30, 2022).

Christina Farr, Health care is one of Apple's most lucrative opportunities: Morgan Stanley. CNBC. 2019. www.cnbc.com/2019/04/08/apple-could-top-300-billion-in-sales-from-health-care-morgan-stanley.html (Accessed on March 30, 2022).

CMS: President Trump Announces Lower Out of Pocket Insulin Costs for Medicare's Seniors May 26, 2020b. https://www.cms.gov/newsroom/press-releases/president-trump-announces-lower-out-pocket-insulin-costs-medicares-seniors (Accessed March 30, 2020).

Commissioner, O. FDA permits marketing of artificial intelligence-based device to detect certain diabetes-related eye problems. 2020; FDA. www.fda.gov/news-events/press-announcements/fda-permits-marketing-artificial-intelligence-based-device-detect-certain-diabetes-related-eye (Accessed on March 30, 2022).

Crown, W.H. Real-World Evidence, Causal Inference, and Machine Learning. Value in Health, 2019; 22(5): 587–592. https://doi.org/10.1016/j.jval.2019.03.001 (Accessed on March 30, 2022).

Dash, S., Shakyawar, S.K., Sharma, M. *et al.* Big data in healthcare: management, analysis and future prospects. *J Big Data* 2019; 6, 54. https://doi.org/10.1186/s40537-019-0217-0. https://journalofbigdata.springeropen.com/articles/10.1186/s40537-019-0217-0#citeas (Accessed on March 30, 2022).

Davenport TH, Dasgupta S. How to Set Up an AI Center of Excellence. Harvard Business Review. 2019. https://hbr.org/2019/01/how-to-set-up-an-ai-center-of-excellence (Accessed on March 30, 2022).

Davis, F.D. Perceived Usefulness, Perceived Ease of Use, and User Acceptance of Information Technology. MIS Quarterly, 1989; 13(3): 319–340. https://doi.org/10.2307/249008 (Accessed on March 30, 2022).

Decencière, E., Zhang, X., Cazuguel, G., Lay, B., Cochener, B., Trone, C., Gain, P., Ordonez, R., Massin, P., Erginay, A., Charton, B. and Klein, J.-C., FEEDBACK ON A PUBLICLY DISTRIBUTED IMAGE DATABASE: THE MESSIDOR DATABASE. Image Analysis & Stereology, 2014; 33(3): 231–234. https://doi.org/10.5566/ias.1155 (Accessed on March 30, 2022).

Digan, W., Neveol, A., Neuraz, A., Wack, M., Baudoin, D., Burgun, A. and Rance, B. Can reproducibility be improved in clinical natural language processing? A study of 7 clinical NLP suites. Journal of the American Medical Informatics Association, 2021; 28(3): 504–515. https://doi.org/10.1093/jamia/ocaa261 (Accessed on March 30, 2022).

Digital Diagnostics. IDx-DR. https://www.digitaldiagnostics.com/products/eye-disease/idx-dr (Accessed on March 30, 2022).

Embedded systems medical and biomedical applications. 2017. https://microcontrollerslab.com/embedded-systems-medical-applications/ (Accessed on March 30, 2022).

Eramo, L.A. Personal Medical Devices: Managing Personal Data, Personally Collected. Journal of AHIMA. 2010; 81: 26–28. http://library.ahima.org/doc?oid=100033 (Accessed on March 30, 2022).

Espay, A.J., Bonato, P., Nahab, F.B., Maetzler, W., Dean, J.M., Klucken, J., Eskofier, B.M., Merola, A., Horak, F., Lang, A.E., Reilmann, R., Giuffrida, J., Nieuwboer, A., Horne, M., Little, M.A., Litvan, I., Simuni, T., Dorsey, E.R., Burack, M.A., Kubota, K., Kamondi, A., Godinho, C., Daneault, J.-F., Mitsi, G., Krinke, L., Hausdorff, J.M., Bloem, B.R. and Papapetropoulos, S., Technology in Parkinson's disease: Challenges and opportunities. Movement Disorders, 2016; 31(9): 1272–1282. https://doi.org/10.1002/mds.26642 (Accessed on March 30, 2022).

Federation of State Medical Boards. U.S. States and Territories Modifying Requirements for Telehealth in Response to COVID-19 (Out-of-state physicians; preexisting provider-patient relationships; audio-only requirements; etc.). 2022. www.fsmb.org/siteassets/advocacy/pdf/states-waiving-licensurerequirements-for-telehealth-in-response-to-covid-19.pdf (Accesssed on March 30, 2022).

Fleming, G.A., Petrie, J.R., Bergenstal, R.M., Holl, R.W., Peters, A.L. and Ford J, Fezza T, Elsner N, Arora A. Key factors to improve drug launches. Deloitte. 2022. www2.deloitte.com/us/en/insights/industry/life-sciences/successful-drug-launch-strategy.html (Accessed on March 30, 2022).

Forcinio, H. Packaging Improves Medication Adherence. Pharmaceutical Technology. 2017; 41: 72–75. https://www.pharmtech.com/view/packaging-improves-medication-adherence (Accessed March 30, 2022).

Ford, K. L., Leiferman, J., Sobral, B., Bennett, J. K., Moore, S. L., & Bull, S. "It depends:" a qualitative study on digital health academic-industry collaboration. mHealth. 2017; 7: 57. https://doi.org/10.21037/mhealth-20-140

Freeman, K., Dinnes, J., Chuchu, N., Takwoingi, Y., Bayliss, S.E., Matin, R.N., Jain, A., Walter, F.M., Williams, H.C. and Deeks, J.J. Algorithm based smartphone apps to assess risk of skin cancer in adults: systematic review of diagnostic accuracy studies. BMJ, [online] 2020; 368: 127. https://doi.org/10.1136/bmj.m127 (Accessed on March 30, 2022).

Fries J.A., Varma P., Chen V.S., et al. Weakly supervised classification of aortic valve malformations using unlabeled cardiac MRI sequences. Nat Commun. 2019;10(1):3111.

FSMB web site, MODEL POLICY FOR THE APPROPRIATE USE OF TELEMEDICINE TECHNOLOGIES IN THE PRACTICE OF MEDICINE April 2014. www.fsmb.org/siteassets/advocacy/policies/fsmb_telemedicine_policy.pdf (Accessed on March 30, 2022).

Gao, F. and Sunyaev, A. Context matters: A review of the determinant factors in the decision to adopt cloud computing in healthcare. International Journal of Information Management. 2019; 48: 120–138. https://doi.org/10.1016/j.ijinfomgt.2019.02.002 2019; 48: 120–138.

Gasser, U. and Almeida, V.A.F. 2017. A Layered Model for AI Governance. IEEE Internet Computing 2017; 21: 58–62. https://doi.org/10.1109/MIC.2017.4180835 (Accessed on March 30, 2022).

Gillespie, L. Telemedicine Policy Draws Opposition From Patient Advocates, Health Care Providers, Kaiser Health News. 2014. https://khn.org/news/telemedicine-policy-draws-opposition-from-patient-advocates (Accessed on March 30, 2022).

Github. Allenai / allennlp-models. 2022. https://github.com/allenai/allennlp-models (Accessed on March 30, 2022).

GitHub. google-research / text-to-text-transfer-transformer. 2022. https://github.com/google-research/text-to-text-transfer-transformer (Accessed on March 30, 2022).

Goodfellow, I.J., Pouget-Abadie, J., Mirza, M., Xu, B., Warde-Farley, D., Ozair, S., Courville, A. and Bengio, Y. Generative Adversarial Networks. arXiv:1406.2661 [cs, stat]. 2014. http://arxiv.org/abs/1406.2661 (Accessed on March 30, 2022).

Gudivada V, Apon A, Ding J. Data quality considerations for big data and machine learning: going beyond data cleaning and transformations. ThinkMind. International Journal on Advances in Software. 2017: 10: 1–20.

Hamrin, V., Sinclair, V.G. and Gardner, V. Theoretical Approaches to Enhancing Motivation for Adherence to Antidepressant Medications. Archives of Psychiatric Nursing. 2017; 31: 223–230. https://doi.org/10.1016/j.apnu.2016.09.004 (Accessed on March 30, 2022).

Habib O. A Quick Primer on Microservices. DZone. 2016. https://dzone.com/articles/a-quick-primer-on-microservices (Accessed on March 30, 2022).

Haenssle HA, Fink C, Schneiderbauer R, Toberer F, Buhl T, Blum A, Kalloo A, Hassen ABH, Thomas L, Enk A, Uhlmann L; Reader study level-I and level-II Groups, Alt C, Arenbergerova M, Bakos R, Baltzer A, Bertlich I, Blum A, Bokor-Billmann T, Bowling J, Braghiroli N, Braun R, Buder-Bakhaya K, Buhl T, Cabo H, Cabrijan L, Cevic N, Classen A, Deltgen D, Fink C, Georgieva I, Hakim-Meibodi LE, Hanner S, Hartmann F, Hartmann J, Haus G, Hoxha E, Karls R, Koga H, Kreusch J, Lallas A, Majenka P, Marghoob A, Massone C, Mekokishvili L, Mestel D, Meyer V, Neuberger A, Nielsen K, Oliviero M, Pampena R, Paoli J, Pawlik E, Rao B, Rendon A, Russo T, Sadek A, Samhaber K, Schneiderbauer R, Schweizer A, Toberer F, Trennheuser L, Vlahova L, Wald A, Winkler J, Wölbing P, Zalaudek I. Man against machine: diagnostic performance of a deep learning convolutional neural network for dermoscopic melanoma recognition in comparison to 58 dermatologists. Ann Oncol. 2018 Aug 1;29(8):1836–1842.

Harrer S, Shah P, Antony B, Hu J. Artificial Intelligence for Clinical Trial Design. Trends Pharmacol Sci. 2019 Aug;40(8):577–591.

Health, C. for D. and R. 2020. Device Software Functions Including Mobile Medical Applications. [online] FDA. www.fda.gov/medical-devices/digital-health-center-excellence/device-software-functions-including-mobile-medical-applications [Accessed on 31 July 2021].

Health, C. for D. and R. Artificial Intelligence and Machine Learning in Software as a Medical Device. FDA. 2021. www.fda.gov/medical-devices/software-medical-device-samd/artificial-intelligence-and-machine-learning-software-medical-device (Accessed on March 30, 2022).

Hogan J. Doctors warn about apps that claim to detect skin cancer. Fox13 Salt Lake City. 2020. https://www.fox13now.com/doctors-warn-about-apps-that-claim-to-detect-skin-cancer (Accessed on March 30, 2022).

Howard, J. and Gugger, S. fastai: A Layered API for Deep Learning. Information, 2020; 11: 108. https://doi.org/10.3390/info11020108 (Accessed on March 30, 2022).

Howard, J. and Ruder, S. Universal Language Model Fine-tuning for Text Classification. arXiv:1801.06146 [cs, stat]. 2018. Available at: http://arxiv.org/abs/1801.06146 (Accessed on March 30, 2022).

IBM Cloud Educations. REST API. 2021. https://www.ibm.com/cloud/learn/rest-apis (Accessed on 30 March 2022).

Iden, J. and Eikebrokk, T.R. Using the ITIL Process Reference Model for Realizing IT Governance: An Empirical Investigation. Information Systems Management, 2014; 31: 37–58. https://doi.org/10.1080/10580530.2014.854089 (Accessed on March 30, 2022).

International Telecommunications Union (ITU). www.itu.int/en/ITU-D/Statistics/Pages/stat/default.aspx World Bank, for population data. https://data.worldbank.org/indicator/SP.POP.TOTL (Accessed on March 30, 2022).

Jackson, G. and Hu, J. Artificial Intelligence in Health in 2018: New Opportunities, Challenges, and Practical Implications. Yearbook of Medical Informatics, 2019; 28(1): 52–54. https://doi.org/10.1055/s-0039-1677925 (Accessed on March 30, 2022).

Janssen, M., Brous, P., Estevez, E., Barbosa, L.S. and Janowski, T. 2020. Data governance: Organizing data for trustworthy Artificial Intelligence. Government Information Quarterly, 2020; 37: 101–493. https://doi.org/10.1016/j.giq.2020.101493 (Accessed on March 30, 2022).

Karale, A. The Challenges of IoT Addressing Security, Ethics, Privacy, and Laws. Internet of Things. 2021; 15: 100–420. https://doi.org/10.1016/j.iot.2021.100420.

Kareem, Z.H., Ramli, K.N. bin, Malik, R.Q. and Zahra, M.M.A. Mobile phone user behavior's recognition using gyroscope sensor and ML algorithms. Materials Today: Proceedings. 2021. https://doi.org/10.1016/j.matpr.2021.04.639 (Accessed on March 30, 2022).

Kashyap A. Artificial Intelligence & Medical Diagnosis. Sch. J. App. Med. Sci. December, 2018; 6(12): 4982–4985.

Khalifa, N.E.M., Loey, M., Taha, M.H.N. and Mohamed, H.N.E.T. Deep Transfer Learning Models for Medical Diabetic Retinopathy Detection. Acta Informatica Medica, 2019; 27(5): 327–332. https://doi.org/10.5455/aim.2019.27.327-332 (Accessed on March 30, 2022).

Khan, A., Sohail, A., Zahoora, U. and Qureshi, A.S. A Survey of the Recent Architectures of Deep Convolutional Neural Networks. Artificial Intelligence Review, 2020; 53(8): 5455–5516. https://doi.org/10.1007/s10462-020-09825-6 (Accessed on March 30, 2022).

Korngiebel, D.M. and Mooney, S.D. Considering the possibilities and pitfalls of Generative Pre-trained Transformer 3 (GPT-3) in healthcare delivery. Npj Digital Medicine, 2021; 4(1): 93. https://doi.org/10.1038/s41746-021-00464-x (Accessed on March 30, 2022).

Krishnakumar, A., Verma, R., Chawla, R., Sosale, A., Saboo, B., Joshi, S., Shaikh, M., Shah, A., Kolwankar, S. and Mattoo, V. Evaluating Glycemic Control in Patients of South Asian Origin With Type 2 Diabetes Using a Digital Therapeutic

Platform: Analysis of Real-World Data. Journal of Medical Internet Research, 2021;23(3): e17908. https://doi.org/10.2196/17908 (Accessed on March 30, 2022).

Kumar, A., Gadag, S. and Nayak, U.Y. The Beginning of a New Era: Artificial Intelligence in Healthcare. Advanced Pharmaceutical Bulletin, 2021; 11(3): 414–425. https://doi.org/10.34172/apb.2021.049 (Accessed on March 30, 2022).

Lee, A.Y., Yanagihara, R.T., Lee, C.S., Blazes, M., Jung, H.C., Chee, Y.E., Gencarella, M.D., Gee, H., Maa, A.Y., Cockerham, G.C., Lynch, M. and Boyko, E.J. Multicenter, Head-to-Head, Real-World Validation Study of Seven Automated Artificial Intelligence Diabetic Retinopathy Screening Systems. Diabetes Care, 2021 44(5): 1168–1175. https://doi.org/10.2337/dc20-1877 (Accessed on March 30, 2022).

Leprince-Ringuet, D. 2021. IBM researchers demonstrate the advantage that quantum computers have over classical computers. [online] ZDNet. Available at: www.zdnet.com/article/ibm-researchers-demonstrate-the-advantage-that-quantum-computers-have-over-classical-computers (Accessed on March 30, 2022).

Lipworth, W. 2019. Real-world Data to Generate Evidence About Healthcare Interventions: The Application of an Ethics Framework for Big Data in Health and Research. Asian Bioethics Review, 2019; 11(3): 289–298. https://doi.org/10.1007/s41649-019-00095-1 (Accessed on March 30, 2022).

Liu X, Faes L, Kale AU, Wagner SK, Fu DJ, Bruynseels A, Mahendiran T, Moraes G, Shamdas M, Kern C, Ledsam JR, Schmid MK, Balaskas K, Topol EJ, Bachmann LM, Keane PA, Denniston AK. A comparison of deep learning performance against health-care professionals in detecting diseases from medical imaging: a systematic review and meta-analysis. Lancet Digit Health. 2019 Oct;1(6):e271–e297.

Lo Piano S. Ethical principles in machine learning and artificial intelligence: cases from the field and possible ways forward. Humanit Soc Sci Commun 2020; 7: 9.

López-Solà M, Woo CW, Pujol J, Deus J, Harrison BJ, Monfort J, Wager TD. Towards a neurophysiological signature for fibromyalgia. Pain. 2017 Jan;158(1):34–47.

Lundervold, A.S. and Lundervold, A. 2019. An overview of deep learning in medical imaging focusing on MRI. Zeitschrift Fur Medizinische Physik. 2019; 29: 102–127. https://doi.org/10.1016/j.zemedi.2018.11.002 (Accessed on March 30, 2022).

Maggsl, 2021. Artificial intelligence (AI) – Azure Architecture Center. https://docs.microsoft.com/en-us/azure/architecture/data-guide/big-data/ai-overview (Accessed on March 30, 2022).

Mäkinen, S., Skogström, H., Laaksonen, E. and Mikkonen, T. Who Needs MLOps: What Data Scientists Seek to Accomplish and How Can MLOps Help? arXiv:2103.08942 [cs]. 2021; http://arxiv.org/abs/2103.08942 (Accessed on March 30, 2022).

Maricich, Y.A., Xiong, X., Gerwien, R., Kuo, A., Velez, F., Imbert, B., Boyer, K., Luderer, H.F., Braun, S. and Williams, K. Real-world evidence for a prescription digital therapeutic to treat opioid use disorder. Current Medical Research and Opinion, 2021; 37: 175–183. https://doi.org/10.1080/03007995.2020.1846023 (Accessed on March 30, 2022).

Martin, A., Andrew Ng Criticizes the Culture of Overfitting in Machine Learning. Unite.AI. 2021; Available at: www.unite.ai/andrew-ng-criticizes-the-culture-of-overfitting-in-machine-learning (Accessed on March 30, 2022).

Martin RD. The Stork-and-Baby Trap. 2013. https://www.psychologytoday.com/us/blog/how-we-do-it/201307/the-stork-and-baby-trap (Accessed on March 30, 2022).

Martinez, K.A., Rood, M., Jhangiani, N. *et al.* Patterns of Use and Correlates of Patient Satisfaction with a Large Nationwide Direct to Consumer Telemedicine Service. *J Gen Intern Med* 2018; 33: 1768–1773 (2018). https://doi.org/10.1007/s11606-018-4621-5 (Accessed on March 30, 2022).

McKinsey. Sustainability. 2020. https://www.mckinsey.com/business-functions/sustainability/how-we-help-clients?cid=alwaysonsus-pse-gaw-mst-mck-oth-2112&gclid=EAIaIQobChMIq9D2jZTv9gIVla_ICh3GQQH1EAAYASAAEgJNR_D_BwE&gclsrc=aw.ds (Accessed on March 30, 2022).

Mehrabi, N., Morstatter, F., Saxena, N., Lerman, K. and Galstyan, A. A Survey on Bias and Fairness in Machine Learning. 2019. arXiv:1908.09635 [cs]. http://arxiv.org/abs/1908.09635 (Accessed on March 30, 2022).

Mehrotra A, Paone S, Martich GD, Albert SM, Shevchik GJ. Characteristics of patients who seek care via eVisits instead of office visits. *Telemed J E Health.* 2013;19(7):515–519. https://pubmed.ncbi.nlm.nih.gov/23682589 (Accessed on March 30, 2022).

Menni, C., Valdes, A.M., Freidin, M.B., Sudre, C.H., Nguyen, L.H., Drew, D.A., Ganesh, S., Varsavsky, T., Cardoso, M.J., El-Sayed Moustafa, J.S., Visconti, A., Hysi, P., Bowyer, R.C.E., Mangino, M., Falchi, M., Wolf, J., Ourselin, S., Chan, A.T., Steves, C.J. and Spector, T.D. Real-time tracking of self-reported symptoms to predict potential COVID-19. Nature Medicine, 2020 26(7): 1037–1040. https://doi.org/10.1038/s41591-020-0916-2 (Accessed on March 30, 2022).

Microcontrollers Lab, Embedded systems medical and biomedical applications. https://microcontrollerslab.com/embedded-systems-medical-applications/.

Mikolov, T., Chen, K., Corrado, G. and Dean, J., Efficient Estimation of Word Representations in Vector Space. arXiv:1301.3781 [cs]. 2013; Available at: http://arxiv.org/abs/1301.3781 (Accessed on March 30, 2022).

Miller, W.R. and Rollnick, S. Motivational Interviewing: Helping People Change. Guilford Press. 2012

Mindfields Global. Artificial intelligence in Healthcare Report. 2018. www.mindfieldsglobal.com/ai-in-healthcare-report (Accessed on March 30, 2022).

Minevich, M. 2021. 5 Steps To Get Digital Enterprises Ready For AI Adoption. [online] Forbes. Available at: www.forbes.com/sites/markminevich/2020/02/19/5-steps-to-get-digital-enterprises-ready-for-ai-adoption/ (Accessed on March 30, 2022).

Morin, C.M. 2020. Profile of Somryst Prescription Digital Therapeutic for Chronic Insomnia: Overview of Safety and Efficacy. Expert Review of Medical Devices, 17(12): 1239–1248. https://doi.org/10.1080/17434440.2020.1852929 (Accessed on March 30, 2022).

Moro, C., Stromberga, Z., Raikos, A. and Stirling, A. The Effectiveness of Virtual and Augmented Reality in Health Sciences and Medical Anatomy. Anatomical Sciences Education, 2017; 10(6): 549–559. https://doi.org/10.1002/ase.1696 (Accessed on March 30, 2022).

Mrozek, D., Koczur, A. and Małysiak-Mrozek, B. Fall detection in older adults with mobile IoT devices and machine learning in the cloud and on the edge. Information Sciences, 2020; 537: 132–147. https://doi.org/10.1016/j.ins.2020.05.070 (Accessed on March 30, 2022).

Neumann, M., King, D., Beltagy, I. and Ammar, W. ScispaCy: Fast and Robust Models for Biomedical Natural Language Processing. In: Proceedings of the 18th BioNLP Workshop and Shared Task. [online] Florence, Italy: Association

for Computational Linguistics. 2019: 319–327. https://doi.org/10.18653/v1/W19-5034 (Accessed on March 30, 2022).
NIST Proposes Approach for Reducing Risk of Bias in Artificial Intelligence, Available at: www.nist.gov/news-events/news/2021/06/nist-proposes-approach-reducing-risk-bias-artificial-intelligence. (Accessed on March 30, 2022).
Nvidia Developer. Deep Learning. 2015. https://developer.nvidia.com/deep-learning (Accessed on March 30, 2022).
Panch T, Mattie H, Atun R. Artificial intelligence and algorithmic bias: implications for health systems. J Glob Health. 2019 Dec;9(2):010318.
Paszke, A., Gross, S., Massa, F., Lerer, A., Bradbury, J., Chanan, G., Killeen, T., Lin, Z., Gimelshein, N., Antiga, L., Desmaison, A., Kopf, A., Yang, E., DeVito, Z., Raison, M., Tejani, A., Chilamkurthy, S., Steiner, B., Fang, L., Bai, J. and Chintala, S. PyTorch: An Imperative Style, High-Performance Deep Learning Library. 2019: 12.
Perry JS. What is big data? More than volume, velocity and variety… IBM Developer. 2017. https://developer.ibm.com/blogs/what-is-big-data-more-than-volume-velocity-and-variety (Accessed on March 30, 2022).
Pew Research Center, www.pewresearch.org/fact-tank/2018/09/28/internet-social-media-use-and-device-ownership-in-u-s-have-plateaued-after-years-of-growth/ (Accessed on March 30, 2022).
Pew Research Center. Chapter 1: Always on Connectivity. 2015. www.pewresearch.org/internet/2015/08/26/chapter-1-always-on-connectivity (Accessed on March 30 2022).
Philip NS, Barredo J, van 't Wout-Frank M, Tyrka AR, Price LH, Carpenter LL. Network Mechanisms of Clinical Response to Transcranial Magnetic Stimulation in Posttraumatic Stress Disorder and Major Depressive Disorder. Biol Psychiatry. 2018 Feb 1;83(3):263–272.
Press release Tufts Center for the Study of Drug Development, New Research from Tufts Center for the Study of Drug Development Characterizes Effectiveness and Variability of Patient Recruitment and Retention Practices (Jan. 15, 2013)
Qayyum A, Qadir J, Bilal M, Al-Fuqaha A. Secure and robust machine learning for healthcare: a survey. IEEE Reviews in Biomedical Engineering. 2021; 14: 156–180.
Raffel, C., Shazeer, N., Roberts, A., Lee, K., Narang, S., Matena, M., Zhou, Y., Li, W. and Liu, P.J. Exploring the Limits of Transfer Learning with a Unified Text-to-Text Transformer. arXiv:1910.10683 [cs, stat]. 2020; http://arxiv.org/abs/1910.10683 (Accessed on March 30, 2022).
Raschka, S., Patterson, J. and Nolet, C. Machine Learning in Python: Main Developments and Technology Trends in Data Science, Machine Learning, and Artificial Intelligence. Information, 2020 11(4): 193. https://doi.org/10.3390/info11040193 (Accessed on March 30, 2022).
Redman TC. Bad data costs the U.S. $3 trillion per year. Harvard Business Review. 2016. https://hbr.org/2016/09/bad-data-costs-the-u-s-3-trillion-per-year (Accessed on March 30, 2022).
Řehůřek, R. and Sojka, P. Software Framework for Topic Modelling with Large Corpora. 2010; University of Malta. Available at: https://is.muni.cz/publication/884893/en/Software-Framework-for-Topic-Modelling-with-Large-Corpora/Rehurek-Sojka (Accessed on March 30, 2022).

Represas-Carrera, F.J., Martínez-Ques, Á.A. and Clavería, A. Effectiveness of mobile applications in diabetic patients' healthy lifestyles: A review of systematic reviews. Primary Care Diabetes. 2021; https://doi.org/10.1016/j.pcd.2021.07.004 (Accessed on March 30, 2022).

Ries, E. The Lean Startup: How Today's Entrepreneurs Use Continuous Innovation to Create Radically Successful Businesses. Illustrated edition ed. 2011; New York: Currency.

Rodriguez, J. 2020. Machine Learning Reference Architectures from Google, Facebook, Uber, DataBricks and Others. DataSeries. https://medium.com/dataseries/machine-learning-reference-architectures-from-google-facebook-uber-databricks-and-others-58191cf82b98 (Accessed on March 30, 2022).

Ryan, R.M. and Deci, E.L. Self-determination theory and the facilitation of intrinsic motivation, social development, and well-being. The American Psychologist, 2000; 55(1): 68–78. https://doi.org/10.1037//0003-066x.55.1.68 (Accessed on March 30, 2022).

Santos, D.F.S., Perkusich, A. and Almeida, H.O. Standard-based and distributed health information sharing for mHealth IoT systems. In: 2014 IEEE 16th International Conference on e-Health Networking, Applications and Services (Healthcom). 2014; 2014 IEEE 16th International Conference on e-Health Networking, Applications and Services (Healthcom 2014). Natal: IEEE. 94–98. https://doi.org/10.1109/HealthCom.2014.7001820 (Accessed on March 30, 2022).

Saunders, M., Lewis, P. and Thornhill, A. Research Methods for Business Students. Prentice Hall. 2009.

Scott, E.M. The role of Statistics in the era of big data: Crucial, critical and undervalued. Statistics & Probability Letters. 2018; 136: 20–24. https://doi.org/10.1016/j.spl.2018.02.050 (Accessed on March 30, 2022).

sdgilley, Architecture & key concepts – Azure Machine Learning. 2021; https://docs.microsoft.com/en-us/azure/machine-learning/concept-azure-machine-learning-architecture (Accessed on March 30, 2022).

Serte, S. and Demirel, H. Deep learning for diagnosis of COVID-19 using 3D CT scans. Computers in Biology and Medicine, 2021; 132): 104306. https://doi.org/10.1016/j.compbiomed.2021.104306 (Accessed on March 30, 2022).

Shaw, J., Rudzicz, F., Jamieson, T. and Goldfarb, A. Artificial Intelligence and the Implementation Challenge. Journal of Medical Internet Research, 2019; 21(7). https://doi.org/10.2196/13659 (Accessed on March 30, 2022).

Singh, T., Bhatnagar, N. and Moond, G.S. Lacunae in noncommunicable disease control program: Need to focus on adherence issues! Journal of Family Medicine and Primary Care. 2017; 6(3): 610–615. https://doi.org/10.4103/2249-4863.21443

spaCy. spaCy 101: Everything you need to know . 2022. https://spacy.io/usage/spacy-101 (Accessed on March 30, 2022).

Skinner, B.F. Operant behavior. American Psychologist, 1963; 18(8): 503–515. https://doi.org/10.1037/h0045185 (Accessed on March 30, 2022).

Statista. LinkedIn's most wanted data science skills in United States as of April 2019. 2022. https://www.statista.com/statistics/1016247/united-states-wanted-data-science-skills (Accessed on March 30, 2022).

Strasser, Kam, and Regalado. Rural Health Care Access and Policy in Developing Countries. Annu. Rev. Public Health 2016; 37:395–412 (Accessed on March 30, 2022).

Sultanow, E., Chircu, A., Schroeder, K. and Kern, S. A Reference Architecture for Pharma, Healthcare & Life Sciences. 2021.

Tamilmani, K., Rana, N.P., Wamba, S.F. and Dwivedi, R. The extended Unified Theory of Acceptance and Use of Technology (UTAUT2): A systematic literature review and theory evaluation. International Journal of Information Management. 2021; (57): 102269. https://doi.org/10.1016/j.ijinfomgt.2020.102269 (Accessed on March 30, 2022).

Tarcar, A.K., Tiwari, A., Dhaimodker, V.N., Rebelo, P., Desai, R. and Rao, D. Healthcare NER Models Using Language Model Pretraining. arXiv:1910.11241 [cs]. 2020 http://arxiv.org/abs/1910.11241 (Accessed on March 30, 2022).

Taulli, T. AI (Artificial Intelligence) Governance: How To Get It Right. [online] Forbes. 2021a. www.forbes.com/sites/tomtaulli/2020/10/10/ai-artificial-intelligence-governance-how-to-get-it-right/ (Accessed on March 30, 2022).

Taulli, T. How To Evaluate AI Software. [online] Forbes. 2021b www.forbes.com/sites/tomtaulli/2021/07/09/how-to-evaluate-ai-software/ (Accessed on March 30, 2022).

TensorFlow. Deploy machine learning models on mobile and edge devices. 2022. https://www.tensorflow.org/lite/ (Accessed on March 30, 2022).

TensorFlow. Pose estimation. 2022. https://www.tensorflow.org/lite/examples/pose_estimation/overview (Accessed on March 30, 2022).

The Open Group. Welcome to the TOGAF® Standard, Version 9.2, a standard of The Open Group. 2022. https://pubs.opengroup.org/architecture/togaf9-doc/arch (Accessed on March 30, 2022).

Thompson, N.C., Greenewald, K., Lee, K. and Manso, G.F. The Computational Limits of Deep Learning. arXiv:2007.05558 [cs, stat]. 2020. http://arxiv.org/abs/2007.05558 (Accessed on March 30, 2022).

Treml C, Genereaux B (Eds.) ACR- AI Lab Hospital Reference Architecture Framework. 2019. https://resources.nvidia.com/en-us-medical-imaging/acr-ai-lab-hospital-architecture-ebook (Accessed on March 30, 2022).

United Nations Department of Social and Economic Affairs (UN DESA) 2021. Our world is growing older: UN DESA releases new report on ageing. Available at: www.un.org/development/desa/en/news/population/our-world-is-growing-older.html (Accessed on March 30, 2022).

US Census Bureau, Computer and Internet Use in the United States: 2015. www.census.gov/content/dam/Census/library/publications/2017/acs/acs-37.pdf.

Verdict, Good Signals from Microcontroller Market. 2020. www.medicaldevice-network.com/features/feature73804/ Microcontrollers Lab (Accessed on March 30, 2022).

Wang, S., Zhang, Y., Lei, S., Zhu, H., Li, J., Wang, Q., Yang, J., Chen, S. and Pan, H. Performance of deep neural network-based artificial intelligence method in diabetic retinopathy screening: a systematic review and meta-analysis of diagnostic test accuracy. European Journal of Endocrinology 2020; 183(1): 41–49. https://doi.org/10.1530/EJE-19-0968 (Accessed on March 30, 2022).

Wang, W., Rothschild, D., Goel, S. and Gelman, A. Forecasting elections with non-representative polls. International Journal of Forecasting 2015; 31(3): 980–991. https://doi.org/10.1016/j.ijforecast.2014.06.001 (Accessed on March 30, 2022).

Waring, J., Lindvall, C. and Umeton, R. Automated machine learning: Review of the state-of-the-art and opportunities for healthcare. Artificial Intelligence in

Medicine. 2020; 104: 101822. https://doi.org/10.1016/j.artmed.2020.101822 (Accessed on March 30, 2022).

Watson, T.F., Philips, S.G.J., Kawakami, E., Ward, D.R., Scarlino, P., Veldhorst, M., Savage, D.E., Lagally, M.G., Friesen, M., Coppersmith, S.N., Eriksson, M.A. and Vandersypen, L.M.K. A programmable two-qubit quantum processor in silicon. Nature. 2018; 555(7698): 633–637. https://doi.org/10.1038/nature25766 (Accessed on March 30, 2022).

Werner R, Emanuel E, Pham HH, Navathe AS. The future of value-based payment: a road map to 2030. Penn LDI, Leonard Davis Institute of Health Economics. 2021. https://ldi.upenn.edu/our-work/research-updates/the-future-of-value-based-payment-a-road-map-to-2030 (Accessed on March 30, 2022).

Wise J. Skin cancer: smartphone diagnostic apps may offer false reassurance, warn dermatologists BMJ 2018; 362 :k2999 doi:10.1136/bmj.k2999

Wilson, H.J. and Daugherty, P.R. 2020. The Next Big Breakthrough in AI Will Be Around Language. Harvard Business Review. [online] 23 Sep. Available at: https://hbr.org/2020/09/the-next-big-breakthrough-in-ai-will-be-around-language (Accessed on March 30, 2022).

World Health Organization. Health workforce. 2020. www.who.int/health-topics/health-workforce (Accessed on March 30, 2022).

World Health Organization. Noncommunicable Diseases. 2022. https://www.who.int/health-topics/noncommunicable-diseases (Accessed July 9, 2022).

Xue, L., Constant, N., Roberts, A., Kale, M., Al-Rfou, R., Siddhant, A., Barua, A. and Raffel, C. 2021. mT5: A massively multilingual pre-trained text-to-text transformer. arXiv:2010.11934 [cs]. [online] Available at: http://arxiv.org/abs/2010.11934 (Accessed on March 30, 2022).

Yi X, Walia E, Babyn P. Generative adversarial network in medical imaging: A review. Med Image Anal. 2019; 58:101552.

Zand A, Sharma A, Stokes Z, Reynolds C, Montilla A, Sauk J, Hommes D. An Exploration Into the Use of a Chatbot for Patients With Inflammatory Bowel Diseases: Retrospective Cohort Study. J Med Internet Res 2020;22(5):e15589.

7

Digital Health Technologies and Innovations

Kelly H. Zou, Mina B. Riad, Shaantanu Donde, Joan van der Horn, and Tarek A. Hassan
Viatris

CONTENTS

7.1 Digital Endpoints and Bring Your Own Device Model

In healthcare, especially in drug development and comparative effectiveness research, there are various types of real-world evidene (RWE) generated from digital sources using health information technology, for example, sensors, monitoring devices, wearables, digital apps, electronic patient-reported outcomes (ePROs), and digital therapeutics (DTx). Such real-world data (RWD) can be big data when vast in quantity and multiple sources are combined (Zou et al., 2020a). In addition, other data sources include genomics, medical imaging, laboratory assays, texts, and physician notes (Zou et al., 2010). More broadly speaking, commonly used data sources to derive insights are insurance and medical claims, electronic health records (EHRs), patient surveys, health risk and status assessments, and patient behaviors and preferences (Capelleri et al., 2013; Alemayehu et al., 2017; Zou et al., 2020c). Methods such as artificial intelligence (AI), machine learning and deep learning are increasingly applied to harness RWD to generate insights

DOI: 10.1201/9781003017523-7

with an impact from end-to-end of research and development, as well as in real-world settings (Katkade et al., 2018; Zou et al., 2020b).

The Food & Drug Administration ([FDA], 2022b) of the United States (US) lists a wide array of digital health technologies that "span a wide range of uses, from applications in general wellness to applications as a medical device," which may be "intended for use as a medical product, in a medical product, as companion diagnostics, or as an adjunct to other medical products (e.g., devices, drugs, and biologics). They may also be used to develop or study medical products."

For example, the 21st Century Cures Act, signed into law in the US on December 13, 2016, has defined real-world evidence (RWE) in Section 3022, where "the term 'real world evidence' means data regarding the usage, or the potential benefits or risks, of a drug derived from sources other than randomized clinical trials" (U.S. Congress, 2016; FDA, 2022b).

The best practices for analysing digital endpoints either in randomized clinical trials (RCTs), pragmatic clinical trials (PCTs) or observational RWE studies depend on the purposes of the studies. For example, "FDA uses RWD and RWE to monitor post market safety and adverse events and to make regulatory decisions. The health care community is using these data to support coverage decisions and to develop guidelines and decision support tools for use in clinical practice. Medical product developers are using RWD and RWE to support clinical trial designs (e.g., large simple trials, pragmatic clinical trials) and observational studies to generate innovative, new treatment approaches" (FDA, 2022b). In addition, the FDA issued a draft guidance on RWD for assessing EHRs and medical claims RWD for regulatory decision-making for drug and biological products (FDA, 2021). Therefore, the purposes of using RWD can be many and varied.

Outside the US, for example, the European Medicine Society (EMA), the United Kingdom (UK) Medicines and Healthcare products Regulatory Agency (MHRA), the Japanese Pharmaceuticals and Medical Device Agency (PMDA), the Chinese National Medical Products Administration (NMPA), and Australian Medicines Australia have also provided definitions and/or issued guidance documents on harnessing RWD to generate RWE for regulatory purposes.

Given such a broad spectrum of usages, it is not only important to identify "fit-for-purpose" data but also endpoints. The Digital Medicine Society (DiMe, 2022) has a rolling repository of digital endpoints, DiMe's Library of Digital Endpoints (2022), which summarize across various features (Table 7.1).

In the context of retrospective observational studies using RWD, FDA (2018) focus on critical questions such as the following:

1. What are the characteristics of the data (e.g., contain data on a relevant endpoint, consistency in documentation, lack of missing data) that improve the chance of a valid result?
2. What are the characteristics of the study design and analysis that improve the chance of a valid result?

TABLE 7.1

DiMe's Library of Digital Endpoints: Entry Fields for Sponsors' Voluntary Entries in Their Original Order of Appearance

1	Date first listed
2	Study phase
3	Endpoint positioning
4	Endpoint (if known)
5	Technology type
6	Health concepts
7	Measurement
8	Indication
9	Sponsor
10	Product type
11	Notes
12	Technology manufacture and device/sensor
13	Analytics company
14	Patient reported outcomes
15	Reference URL
16	Sponsor and/or principal investigator (PI) contact
17	Publications
18	Date of addiction

(a) Can an active comparator improve the chance of a valid result?
(b) Given potential unmeasured confounders in non-randomized RWD studies, as well as potential measurement variability in RWD, is there a role for non-inferiority designs?

3. What sensitivity analyses and statistical diagnostics should be prespecified for observational studies using RWD to generate RWE for effectiveness?

When considering the studies with digital endpoints, there are various types: randomized controlled trials, non-interventional observational studies, and a hybrid, which is a pragmatic clinical trial.

First, RCT is a study in which randomization is used to assign patients to multiple treatments. The purpose of an RCT is to: (1) to guard against any use of judgment or systematic arrangements leading to one treatment getting preferential assignment, i.e., to avoid bias; (2) to provide a basis for the standard methods of statistical analysis such as significance tests. See: FDA (2022c). It is another term for an interventional study. See: U.S. National Library of Medicine (2021).

Second, observational study is a type of study in which individuals are observed or certain outcomes are measured. No attempt is made to affect the outcome (for example, no treatment is given). See: National Cancer Institute (2021). Thus, it tends to be non-interventional.

Third, Pragmatic Clinical Trial (PCT) is those clinical trials for which the hypothesis and study design are developed specifically to answer the questions faced by decision makers, and they are either pragmatic or practical. The characteristic features of PCTs are that they (1) select clinically relevant alternative interventions to compare, (2) include a diverse population of study participants, (3) recruit participants from heterogeneous practice settings, and (4) collect data on a broad range of health outcomes. See: Tunis et al. (2003).

There are best practices for each of the above types of studies, and checklists are also of a useful approach to implementing such practices (Table 7.2).

Now, in a hypothetical example, let's consider the bring Your Own Device (BYOD) model in a study. To facilitate patients' engagement, improve interaction, and potentially increase adherence, BYOD utilizes devices such as

TABLE 7.2

Best Practices and Checklists by Study Type

Study Type	Good Practices	Checklist
Randomized Controlled Trials	1. RCTs should be planned from the beginning of the program 2. RCTs need a large sample size 3. RCTs should be undertaken following formative research or evaluation 4. RCTs must be appropriate to the nature of the program being assessed (See: White et al., 2014.)	The CONSORT (CONsolidated Standards of Reporting Trials) 2010 guideline is intended to improve the reporting of parallel group RCT, enabling readers to understand an RCT's design, conduct, analysis, and interpretation, and to assess the validity of its results. This can only be achieved through complete adherence and transparency by authors. (See CONSORT, 2021; Schulz et al., 2010)
Pragmatic Clinical Trials	Key design elements: 1. Real-world population 2. Real-world setting 3. Appropriate comparator arm 4. Relevant outcome Considerations for bias reduction: 1. Hard endpoints 2. Adjudication by blinded medical experts 3. Trial conduct, statistical analysis plan development and beyond by blinded statistician or data analyst (See: Gamerman et al., 2019)	The CONSORT extension for pragmatic trials builds upon the existing CONSORT checklist and gives specific guidance for 8 of the 22 checklist items in relation to pragmatic trials. (See CONSORT, 2021; Zwarenstein et al., 2008)

TABLE 7.2 Continued

Best Practices and Checklists by Study Type

Study Type	Good Practices	Checklist
Observational Non-Interventional Studies	The overall aims of this Observational CER User's Guide for the design of such protocols are to identify both minimal standards and best practices for designing observational CER studies in the DEcIDE Network. Evidence is generally considered strong when appraised studies show consistent results, are well designed to minimize bias, and are from representative patient populations. (See: Velentgas et al., 2013.) The International Society for Pharmacoeconomics and Outcomes Research (ISPOR) and the International Society for Pharmacoepidemiology (ISPE) created a task force to make recommendations regarding good procedural practices that would enhance decision makers' confidence in evidence derived from RWE studies. (See: Berger et al., 2017.) Designed as a set of high-level questions, the Good ReseArch for Comparative Effectiveness GRACE Principles lay out the elements of good practice for the design, conduct, analysis, and reporting of observational CER studies. (See: GRACE, 2021; Dreyer et al., 2010.)	STaRT-RWE is a structured template for planning and reporting on the implementation of real-world evidence studies. The template serves as a guiding tool for designing and conducting reproducible RWE studies; set clear expectations for transparent communication of RWE methods; reduce misinterpretation of prose that lacks specificity; allow reviewers to quickly orient and find key information; and facilitate reproducibility, validity assessment, and evidence synthesis. (See: Wang et al., 2021.) The GRACE initiative provides guidance to enhance the quality of observational comparative effectiveness research (CER) and a checklist to facilitate its use for decision support. (See: GRACE, 2021; Dreyer et al., 2014; Dreyer et al. 2016.)

mobile phone devices, sensors, watches, is increasingly useful and adopted. Often, the methodology of collecting data via mobile phone applications can be ePROs, which can be digitization rather than DTx, and increasingly, the QR code technology can be applied (Pugliese, 2010).

The advantages are timely interaction, user friendliness, and easy access, without adding extra trial setup cost by providing a designated device. The potential limitations can be phone app updates, internet WiFi availability and signal strength, and device-access persistently and consistently.

In the BYOD applications, the standard methods for a PCT may be adopted, where the intervention arms are via remote monitoring and digital therapeutics: (1) a BYOD arm with a specific mobile app for medication dosage monitoring and usage via ePRO-capture, vs. (2) a usual care arm without this specific mobile app. These two interventional arms are considered mutually exclusive. However, in practice, patients under usual care increasingly have access to mobile devices like smart phones, especially given reduced mobility and clinic visits during the COVID-19 pandemic.

There are several key factors to consider as best practices when designing the study, developing its protocol and statistical analysis plan (SAP), as in Table 7.2 for PCTs. Potentially, biases can occur for the following reasons:

(1) Confounder due to non-mutually exclusive groups between the two arms in terms of other apps that could function in a similar way.
(2) Unmet need due to the lack of access to Wi-Fi and mobile device, particularly for elderly patients or those from underrepresented populations.
(3) Missing data due to lack of signal during real-time monitoring, e.g., when patients are on a subway without reliable Wi-Fi signal.
(4) Properties of PRO instrument and validation; see, e.g., FDA's (2009) final PRO guidance for use in RCTs, and similarly in PCTs; also see: Cappelleri (2013).
(5) Statistical considerations and methods such as sample size calculation, minimal clinical important difference, correlation, univariate and multivariate analyses, and predictive model, depending on the type of primary, secondary and exploratory endpoints or outcome variables that can be either discrete or continuous; see, e.g., Zou et al. (2003a; 2003b; 2007); Alemayehu et al. (2017); product and process comparisons with formulae via the U.S. National Institute of Standards and Technology (2021).
(6) Appropriate methods explore the association or causal relationship between the baseline variables such as patient characteristics, comorbid conditions that can be risk factors, intervention arms, and the endpoints such as medication use, adherence and persistence; see: Alemayehu et al. (2017).
(7) Sophisticated methods may be applicable to digital data, e.g., artificial intelligence is the science and engineering of making intelligent machines, especially intelligent computer programs; machine learning is a system that has the capacity to learn based on training on a specific task by tracking performance measures; deep learning is a subset of machine learning, applies algorithms using an artificial neural network comprising layered connections. These connections evaluate and process input data to yield a desired output classification (Zou et al., 2020b).

(8) Human subject protection, patient consent, intuitional review board (IRB) in the US or ethics committees in the EU for approvals, data privacy, and ethical conducts (Cohen et al., 2018).

7.2 Wearables and Sensors

Wearables and sensors are challenging and changing the healthcare system by allowing patients to monitor their vitals outside the hospitals or medical facility, they can give continuous real time data giving patients clear insights about their overall condition, diseases or even for fitness purposes (Dunn et al., 2018; Kim et al., 2019).

Medical wearables are electronic devices that consumers can wear, designed to collect the data of users' personal health. They can be an integral part of personal analytics, measuring physical status, recording physiological parameters. For instant, hearing aids, pulse, oxygen levels, airflow, body temperature, skin response, continuous glucose monitoring (CGM), ECG, blood pressure monitoring, etc. (Business Insider 2021).

Sensors are the tools that detect physical, chemical, and biological signals providing a way for those signals to be measured and recorded for e.g., smart pacemakers, artificial retinas, and chemical sensors. The medical staff will obtain information online about a patient's blood chemistries, electrocardiogram, blood pressure, and temperature. A diabetic patient will have a smart glucose sensor or insulin reservoir system implanted or even a continuous glucose monitoring (CGM) system. Not only for adults but also sensors now can measure vitals for fetus like heart rate during labor or monitor the lactate in their blood (Wilson, 1999 and Cummins et al., 2018).

Combining wearables and sensors together allows researchers to reach new heights of digital innovations, from sensing patients' biological data and monitoring them, to conducting real-time analysis. Patients can now monitor their heart rate, ECG, blood oxygen saturation all in one device. Diabetic patients can have continuous glucose monitoring with real-time data via medical charts for analysis (Ray et al., 2020). The future and the competition in smart healthcare are on combining sensors and wearables in one device. Doctors and nurses will have real-time data in high frequencies, without extensive research or diagnosis. Patients with Parkinsonism can have real time brain stimulation, pacemakers will protect from heart attacks. Patients will be warned about a danger from any health issue happening to their hearts or brains and these devices can even seek help for them (Hagargi and Kumbhar, 2020).

RWD can be gathered immediately out of wearables and sensors (Kim et al., 2019). They can jointly be used to collect RWD for a clear diagnosis. Patients do not need to visit their doctors, but instead speak on the phone with them or schedule a tele-visit and the facility will ship sensors and devices to collect health data from the patients (Tuominen et al., 2019).

7.3 Digital Therapeutics and Apps

Digital technologies have long impacted the field of health. From the 1970s, the expanding availability of personal computers allowed health data to be increasingly digitized and centralized in local, national, and more recently global databases (Lupton and Maslen, 2017).

Digital health is a broad umbrella word that includes both digital medicine and DTx. Technology, processes, and platforms that engage "consumers" to maintain their lifestyle and wellness are referred to as digital health. Clinical operations and life sciences are supported by some digital health applications. Examples include wellness apps, telehealth, and clinical care administration and management tools.

Clinical evidence is not usually required for digital health applications. However, evidence-based software or hardware products are typically used in digital medicine applications to assess (diagnose) or intervene. Regulatory approval is required for digital medicine goods that are classified as "medical devices." Examples include digital diagnostics, remote patient monitoring software, and decision-support software (Digital Therapeutic Alliance, 2019).

DTx is different from both digital health and digital medicine in that DTx comprises evidence-based "interventions" designed for the purpose of preventing, managing, or treating a particular disorder or health condition. In other words, DTx is like a digital pill, which requires a similar level of clinical and real-world evidence, regulatory oversight, and clearance as it is required for conventional pharmaceutical products (White Paper: Digital Therapeutics). Thus, DTx products are not merely "wellness apps" but are evidence-based specific interventions delivered digitally.

DTx is a digital health category defined by the Digital Therapeutics Alliance as products that "deliver evidence-based therapeutic interventions to patients that are driven by high quality software programs to prevent, manage, or treat a medical disorder or disease" (Digital Therapeutics Alliance, 2021).

Mobile health (mHealth), along with DTx, becomes widely accepted as necessary for the future of efficient healthcare service delivery. Significant advances in computing power, access to smart devices, and connectivity over the last decade, have given rise to an entire industry capable of transforming the way healthcare is delivered. These digital health solutions have the potential to expand access to care and enhance our understanding of populations, pathology and how services can be improved for patients and service users at scale.

Advances in and the increasingly dominant role of mobile technology and AI in our everyday lives have broadened the role of DTx in healthcare. When compared to standard pharmacological interventions alone, this new innovation will raise patients' awareness of their health and their ability to take a more active role in controlling their disease, perhaps improving health outcomes and reducing demands on healthcare systems (Chung, 2019).

The DTx market is expected to grow tenfold in the next three to five years, with a projected market value of $9 billion (USD) by 2025. (See: White Paper: Digital Therapeutics: Past Trends and Future Prospects, 2021). However, this presents challenges in terms of how the technology is regulated, how healthcare providers (HCPs) may respond to this paradigm shift, and how these technologies are reimbursed. Magnetic resonance (MR) imaging and computed tomography (CT)scanners, EHRs with physicians' notes, e-prescriptions, and pacemakers are just a few examples of technological progress in healthcare. A growing number of businesses are focusing on using digital tools to improve the quality and accessibility of care, particularly for chronic illnesses, which account for a significant portion of rising healthcare expenses. During the coronavirus disease 2019 (COVID-19) pandemic, quarantines and lockdowns might make services like telemedicine and online patient monitoring the only means to get medical or mental health care in many circumstances, therefore the pandemic has raised the patients' and caregivers' demand for these products (Tang et al., 2019; Feingold et al., 2019).

With respect to therapeutic areas, for example, the highest percentage of trials have been conducted in psychiatric indications (25%). There is strong evidence supporting digital cognitive behavior therapy's (DCBT) efficacy in this area, followed by cardiovascular (11%), endocrine (10%), addiction (10%), neurology (8%), and respiratory (7%). Seventy-seven percent of DTx trials conducted over the past ten years have been sponsored by academia, which has dominated research across all TAs apart from respiratory, where 50% of trials have been sponsored by industry. Although traditional cognitive behavior therapy (CBT) has been effective in improving health outcomes in chronic nephrology and gastroenterology indications, there has been very little research to investigate the effectiveness of digital modalities in these TAs (Ng et al., 2019; Feingold et al., 2019).

Digital health tools include various technologies that can enhance health and health service delivery. Such tools can range from instruments that improve communication between healthcare providers and patients, e.g., telemedicine technology, to EHRs, mobile apps for monitoring symptoms, and medication and appointment reminder systems. These tools have been used for a range of purposes during the COVID-19 pandemic, including telemedicine service provision; remote patient monitoring; digital communication between political leaders and scientific authorities; and digital data-monitoring to track COVID-19 spread, COVID-19 evolution, and people's perceptions. However, most countries lack a regulatory framework to authorize, integrate, and reimburse telemedicine services, and there is large heterogeneity between countries (Monaco et al., 2021).

7.4 Remote Patient Monitoring

According to the FDA (2022a), "digital technology has been driving a revolution in health care. Digital health tools have the vast potential to improve our ability to accurately diagnose and treat disease and to enhance the delivery of health care for the individual." We have shed some light on digital health technologies, which are evolving constantly and rapidly. Given the vast array of applications, protecting patient privacy, making technologies validated and transparent, while encouraging health innovations can be a balancing act that would need multi-stakeholder collaborations between the healthcare and technology sectors.

Nowadays, comprehensive medical care, and the use of technology in the healthcare field have been substantially growing especially with the increase in the aging population and noncommunicable diseases (NCDs) around the world (Malasinghe et al., 2019).

Telehealth is

> a mode of delivering health care services and public health via information and communication technologies to facilitate the diagnosis, consultation, treatment, education, care management, and self-management of a patient's health care while the patient is at the originating site and the health care provider is at a distant site.
>
> California Business and Professions Code

Telemedicine is "the ability of physicians and patients to connect via technology other than through virtual interactive physician/patient capabilities, especially enabling rural and out of-area patients to be seen by specialists remotely" (California Code of Regulation).

Home-based patient monitoring and follow up is an emerging healthcare field as we move towards using new digital technology in the form of sensors and smart devices to remotely monitor patients and inform their healthcare providers about their illnesses and measure their progress with treatment (Bayoumy et al., 2021).

Remote patient monitoring, (e.g., telehealth, mHealth) help in keeping patients outside hospitals and protect the fragile and immunocompromised from acquiring nosocomial infections especially during the fulminant times in the pandemic (Clinical Management of COVID-19).

The United States Government Accountability Office (GAO) defined in their Report to Congressional Committees, the remote patient monitoring as the technology to enable monitoring of patients outside of conventional clinical settings, such as in the home (GAO, 2022).

Also, the GAO stated that remote patient monitoring can be used to monitor patients with chronic conditions, such as those with congestive heart failure, hypertension, diabetes mellitus, and chronic obstructive pulmonary disease. It can also be used as a diagnostic tool, such as for some heart conditions (GAO, 2017).

The U.S. Department of Health and Human Services (HHS) has found that the most consistent benefit of telehealth and remote patient monitoring occurs when the technology is used for communication and counseling or to remotely monitor chronic conditions such as cardiovascular and respiratory diseases, with improvements in outcomes such as mortality, quality of life, and reductions in hospital admissions (GAO, 2017).

The remote patient monitoring (RPM) modality collects patient information electronically and transmits it to a provider at another location to allow tracking and monitoring of that patient. Common RPMs include glucose and blood pressure monitoring. This type of remote patient monitoring is critical, as the industry moves toward pay-for-performance and reimbursement methods. In addition, RPMs may assist hospitals in monitoring newly released patients in an effort to prevent readmissions from complications after discharge. Chronic conditions are well serviced by RPM as well. For example, the Veterans Administration (VA), one of the largest users of RPM services, reported that its Care Coordination/Home Telehealth program monitored and cared for more than 70,000 veterans with chronic diseases in 2012, and that patient satisfaction levels were greater than 85%. The VA also reported more than $9,000 in savings per patient due to the reduction in the number of hospitalizations (Marcoux and Vogenberg 2016).

Remarks

The center of digital health technologies and innovations are the patients and other multiple stakeholders. In "tech," the speed to market and mass-adoptions may be critical, as in the smart device industry. However, in healthcare, since it is a highly regulated industry, the hurdle for "health tech" is greater due to the specialty therapeutic knowledge, experience and practice. Therefore, for such technologies to thrive, where patients not only adhere to their therapies, but also maintain an interest in adhering to these smart tools, may be challenging.

Nevertheless, given the fact that the COVID-19 pandemic has enabled the healthcare industry to think creatively to engage their patients and caregivers via eHealth, mHealth, and telehealth, as well as through smart trials, pragmatic studies, observational studies, as well as remote patient monitoring, the digital world may well intersect with the real world to generate comprehensive RWE from RWD through innovative applications as use case.

Disclaimer

Kelly H. Zou, Shaantanu Donde, Joan van der Horn and Tarek A. Hassan are employees of Viatris, merged between Upjohn, a Division of Pfizer, and Mylan. Mina B. Riad is a former contractor of Upjohn, a Division of Pfizer, and Viatris. The views expressed are the authors' own and do not necessarily represent those of their employer or employers. The authors appreciate the editorial support from Arghya Bhattacharya and Aswin Kumar A of Viatris.

References

Alemayehu D, Cappelleri JC, Emir B, Zou KH. Statistical Topics in HEOR. Boca Raton, FL: Taylor & Francis, 2017.

Bayoumy K, Gaber M, Elshafeey A, Mhaimeed O, Dineen EH, Marvel FA, Martin SS, Muse ED, Turakhia MP, Tarakji KG, Elshazly MB. Smart wearable devices in cardiovascular care: where we are and how to move forward. Nat. Rev. Cardiol. 2021; 1–19.

Berger ML, Sox H, Willke RJ et al. Good Practices for Real-World Data Studies of Treatment and/or Comparative Effectiveness: Recommendations from the Joint ISPOR-ISPE Special Task Force on Real-World Evidence in Health Care Decision Making. Value Health. 2017; 20(8): 1003–1008.

California Business and Professions Code (BPC) Section 2290.5 (e)

California Code of Regulation Title 10 Section 6410

Cappelleri JC, Zou KH et al. PROs: From Measurement to Interpretation. London, UK: Chapman & Hall/CRC Press, Taylor & Francis Group, 2013.

Chung JY. Digital Therapeutics and Clinical Pharmacology. Transl Clin Pharmacol. 2019 Mar; 27(1): 6–11

Cohen IG, Lynch HF, Vayena E, Gasser U (eds). Big Data, Health Law, and Bioethics. Cambridge University Press; 1st edition. New York, NY; Cambridge: Cambridge University Press, 2018.

CONSORT – CONsolidated Standards Of Reporting Trials. About CONSORT. 2010. www.consort-statement.org/about-consort (Accessed March 30, 2022).

Cummins G, Kremer J, Bernassau A, Brown A, Bridle HL, Schulze H, Bachmann TT, Crichton M, Denison FC, Desmulliez MP. Sensors for fetal hypoxia and metabolic acidosis: a review. Sensors. 2018; 18(8): 2648

Digital therapeutic alliance Digital Health, Digital Medicine, Digital Therapeutics (DTx): What's the difference? 2020. https://dtxalliance.org (Accessed March 30, 2022).

DiMe's Library of digital endpoints. 2022. www.dimesociety.org/index.php/knowledge-center/library-of-digital-endpoints (Accessed March 30, 2022).

DoD COVID-19 PRACTICE MANAGEMENT GUIDE Clinical Management of COVID-19 https://apps.dtic.mil/sti/pdfs/AD1097348.pdf (Accessed March 30, 2022).

Dreyer NA, Bryant A, Velentgas P. The GRACE Checklist: A Validated Assessment Tool for High Quality Observational Studies of Comparative Effectiveness. J. Managed Care Spec. Pharm. 2016; 22(10): 1107–13.

Dreyer NA, Schneeweiss S, McNeil B, et al. GRACE Principles: Recognizing high-quality observational studies of comparative effectiveness. Am. J. Managed Care. 2010; 16(6): 467–471.

Dreyer NA, Velentgas P, Westrich K et al. The GRACE Checklist for Rating the Quality of Observational Studies of Comparative Effectiveness: A Tale of Hope and Caution. J. Managed Care Pharm.. 2014; 20(3): 301–08.

Dunn J, Runge R, Snyder M. Wearables and the medical revolution. Pers. Med. 2018; 15(5): 429–448

Enhanced Patient-Centricity: Optimizing Patient Care Through AI/ML/DL www.pharmavoice.com/wp-content/uploads/PV0620_EnhancedPatientCentricity_WM.pdf?tracker_id=1594684800202 (Accessed March 30, 2022).

Feingold J, Murray HB, Keefer L. Recent Advances in Cognitive Behavioral Therapy for Digestive Disorders and the Role of Applied Positive Psychology Across the Spectrum of GI Care. J. Clin. Gastroenterol. 2019 Aug;53(7):477–485

Food & Drug Administration. Framework for FDA's real-world evidence program. 2018. www.fda.gov/media/120060/download (Accessed March 30, 2022).

Food & Drug Administration. Glossary of terms on clinical trials for patient engagement advisory committee meeting. 2022c. www.fda.gov/media/108378/download (Accessed March 30, 2022).

Food & Drug Administration. Patient-Reported Outcome Measures: Use in Medical Product Development to Support Labeling Claims: Guidance for Industry. 2009. www.fda.gov/regulatory-information/search-fda-guidance-documents/patient-reported-outcome-measures-use-medical-product-development-support-labeling-claims (Accessed March 30, 2022).

Food & Drug Administration. Real-World Data: Assessing Electronic Health Records and Medical Claims Data to Support Regulatory Decision-Making for Drug and Biological Products. 2021. www.fda.gov/regulatory-information/search-fda-guidance-documents/real-world-data-assessing-electronic-health-records-and-medical-claims-data-support-regulatory (Accessed March 30, 2022).

Food & Drug Administration. Real-world evidence. 2022b. www.fda.gov/science-research/science-and-research-special-topics/real-world-evidence (Accessed March 30, 2022).

Food & Drug Administration. What is Digital Health? 2022a. www.fda.gov/medical-devices/digital-health-center-excellence/what-digital-health (Accessed March 30, 2022).

Gamerman V, Cai T, Elsäßer A. Pragmatic randomized clinical trials: best practices and statistical guidance. Health Serv. Outcomes Res. Methodol. 2019; 19: 23–35.

Getting real with wearable data. Editorial. Nat Biotechnol. 2019; 37: 331. https://doi.org/10.1038/s41587-019-0109-z (Accessed March 30, 2022).

Government Accountability Office. Telehealth and Remote Patient Monitoring Use in Medicare and Selected Federal Programs. Health Care: Telehealth and Remote Patient Monitoring Use in Medicare and Selected Federal Programs. 2017. www.gao.gov/products/gao-17-365 (Accessed March 30, 2022).

GRACE. Good ReseArch for Comparative Effectiveness. 2021. www.graceprinciples.org/grace.html (Accessed March 30, 2022).

Hagargi PA, Kumbhar S. Combined Effects of IoTs and Medical Sensors for Effective Application of Smart HealthCare System. J. Eng., Comput. and Archit. 2020; 10(4): 11–19

J Med Internet Res. 2021; 23(1): e25652. doi: 10.2196/25652

Katkade VB, Sanders KN, Zou KH. Real world data: an opportunity to supplement existing evidence for the use of long-established medicines in health care decision making. J Multidiscip Healthc. 2018 Jul 2; 11: 295–304.

Kim J, Campbell AS, de Ávila BEF, Wang J. Wearable biosensors for healthcare monitoring. Nat. Biotechnol. 2019; 37: 389–406.

Latest trends in medical monitoring devices and wearable health technology www.businessinsider.com/wearable-technology-healthcare-medical-devices#:~:text=What%20is%20wearable%20healthcare%20technology,users%27%20personal%20health%20and%20exercise.(Accessed March 30, 2022).

Lupton D, Maslen S. Telemedicine and the senses: a review. Sociol Health Illn. 2017 Nov; 39(8): 1557–1571.

Malasinghe LP, Ramzan N, Dahal K. Remote patient monitoring: a comprehensive study. J. Ambient Intell. and Humanized Comput. 2019; 10(1), 57–76.

Marcoux RM, Vogenberg FR. Telehealth: applications from a legal and regulatory perspective. Pharm Ther. 2016; 41(9): 567.

National Cancer Institute, National Institutes of Health. Observational study. 2021. www.cancer.gov/publications/dictionaries/cancer-terms/def/observational-study (Accessed March 30, 2022).

National Institute of Standards and Technology. 2021. www.itl.nist.gov/div898/handbook/index.htm (Accessed March 30, 2022).

National Library of Medicine. ClinicalTrials.gov. 2021. https://clinicaltrials.gov/ct2/about-studies/glossary (Accessed March 30, 2022).

Ng CZ, Tang SC, Chan M et al. A Systematic Review and Meta-Analysis of Randomized Controlled Trials of Cognitive Behavioral Therapy for Hemodialysis Patients with Depression. J Psychosom Res. 2019 Nov

Pugliese L, Woodriff M, Crowley O, Lam V, Sohn J, Bradley S. Feasibility of the "Bring Your Own Device" Model in Clinical Research: Results from a Randomized Controlled Pilot Study of a Mobile Patient Engagement Tool. Cureus. 2016 Mar 16; 8(3): e535.

Ray PP, Dash D, Kumar N. Sensors for internet of medical things: State-of-the-art, security and privacy issues, challenges and future directions. Comput. Commun. 2020; 160: 111–131.

Schulz KF, Altman DG, Moher D; CONSORT Group. CONSORT 2010 statement: updated guidelines for reporting parallel group randomized trials. BMJ. 2010 Mar 23; 340: c332.

Steinhubl SR, Muse ED, Topol EJ. The emerging field of mobile health. Sci Transl Med. 2015; 7: 283rv3.

Transforming Global Healthcare by Advancing Digital Therapeutics Available at: https://dtxalliance.org Accessed March 30, 2022).

Tunis SR, Stryer DB, Clancy CM. Practical clinical trials: increasing the value of clinical research for decision making in clinical and health policy. JAMA. 2003 Sep 24; 290(12): 1624–32.

Tuominen J, Peltola K, Saaresranta T, Valli K. Sleep parameter assessment accuracy of a consumer home sleep monitoring ballistocardiograph beddit sleep tracker: a validation study. J. Clin. Sleep Med. 2019; 15(3): 483–487.

U.S. Congress, H.R.34 – 21st Century Cures Act. Washington DC. 2016. www.congress.gov/bill/114th-congress/house-bill/34 (Accessed March 30, 2022).

Velentgas P, Dreyer NA, Nourjah P, Smith SR, Torchia MM (eds). Developing a Protocol for Observational Comparative Effectiveness Research: A User's Guide. AHRQ Publication No. 12(13)-EHC099. Rockville, MD: Agency for Healthcare Research and Quality, 2013. https://effectivehealthcare.ahrq.gov/sites/default/files/related_files/user-guide-observational-cer-130113.pdf (Accessed March 30, 2022).

Wang SV, Pinheiro S, Hua W, Arlett P, Uyama Y, Berlin JA, Bartels DB, Kahler KH, Bessette LG, Schneeweiss S. STaRT-RWE: structured template for planning and reporting on the implementation of real world evidence studies. BMJ. 2021 Jan 12; 372: m4856.

White H, Sabarwal S, de Hoop T. Randomized Controlled Trials (RCTs): Methodological Briefs – Impact Evaluation No. 7, Methodological Briefs no. 7. 2014. www.unicef-irc.org/publications/752-randomized-controlled-trials-rcts-methodological-briefs-impact-evaluation-no-7.html (Accessed March 30, 2022).

White Paper: Digital Therapeutics: Past Trends and Future Prospects – Evidera. [online] Available at: www.evidera.com/digital-therapeutics-past-trends-and-future-prospects (Accessed March 30, 2022).

Wilson CB. Sensors in medicine. BMJ. 1999; 319(7220): 1288

Zou KH, Fielding JR, Silverman SG, Tempany CM. Hypothesis testing I: proportions. Radiology. 2003a Mar; 226(3): 609–613

Zou KH, Li JZ, Imperato J, Potkar CN, Sethi N, Edwards J, Ray A. Harnessing Real-World Data for Regulatory Use and Applying Innovative Applications. J Multidiscip Healthc. 2020a; 13: 671–679.

Zou KH, Li JZ, Ovalle J, Li, Seth N, Ray A. Optimizing Patient Care Through AI/ML/DL. PharmaVoice. 2020b June.

Zou KH, Li JZ, Salem LA, Imperato J, et al. Harnessing real-world evidence to reduce the burden of noncommunicable disease: health information technology and innovation to generate insights. Health Serv. Outcomes Res. Methodol. 2020c: 1–13.

Zou KH, Liu A, Bandos AI, Ohno-Machado L, Rochette HE. Statistical Evaluation of Diagnostic Performance: Topics in ROC Analysis. London: Taylor & Francis Group, 2010.

Zou KH, O'Malley AJ, Mauri L. Receiver-operating characteristic analysis for evaluating diagnostic tests and predictive models. Circulation. 2007 Feb 6; 115(5): 654–657.

Zou KH, Tuncali K, Silverman SG. Correlation and simple linear regression. Radiology. 2003b Jun; 227(3): 617–622.

Zwarenstein M, Treweek S, Gagnier JJ, Altman DG, Tunis S, Haynes B, Oxman AD, Moher D; CONSORT group; Pragmatic Trials in Healthcare (Practihc) group. Improving the reporting of pragmatic trials: an extension of the CONSORT statement. BMJ. 2008 Nov 11; 337: a2390.

8

Economic Analysis and Outcome Assessment

Jean-Pascal Roussy and Kelly H. Zou
Viatris

CONTENTS

8.1 Economic Analysis

The scientific progress and development of new health technologies (e.g., medications, medical devices, and medical procedures) contribute to advancing patient care and outcomes. With the aging of societies in the developed economies and a demographic boom in lower- and middle-income countries (LMICs), healthcare is expected to continue to play a pivotal role in keeping populations healthy and active. However, the increasing demand for services and the resulting pressure on medical expenditures confront payers, drug plan managers, hospital administrators and other public and private decision makers with challenging budget allocation decisions. With scarce resources, it is paramount to use a robust and evidence-based approach to identify the health technologies that will deliver the best value for money. This approach is usually referred to as health technology assessment (HTA). We will review how the economic evaluations, a core constituent of the HTA process, can support value determination and adoption of novel heath technologies, and also briefly explore the role of patients in these assessments.

In the health sector, different types of economic evaluations can be conducted. To understand the economic burden of a disease to society, cost-of-illness studies are performed. Those capture all direct and non-direct

DOI: 10.1201/9781003017523-8

TABLE 8.1

Overview of Economic Evaluation, by Type

Type of Analysis	Description	Valuation of Costs (for All Analyses)	Valuation of Consequences	Composite Measure of Value
Cost-of-illness studies (COI)	• Describe the economic burden of a disease to society • Does not compare health technologies	• Health care perspective: direct and indirect medical costs • Societal perspective: direct and indirect medical costs, non-medical costs • Direct medical costs: e.g., medications, medical procedures, laboratory tests • Non-direct medical costs: e.g., patient-time costs, unpaid caregiver-time costs, transportation costs • Non-Medical costs: e.g., productivity, consumption, social services, legal or criminal justice, education, housing, environment	• Medical consequences (longevity, morbidity) • Non-medical consequences	• NA
Cost-minimization analysis (CMA)	• Assumes similar effectiveness between the technologies studied • Examines only the cost related to each technology • Favored the technology associated with the lowest cost	• As above	• NA	• NA

Cost-consequence analysis (CCA)	• Lists all costs and consequences related to the studied technologies • Disaggregated results: offer transparency	• As above	• Medical consequences (longevity, morbidity) • Non-medical consequences	• NA
Cost-effectiveness analyses (CEA)	• Compares the cost and consequences of two technologies • Generate a composite measure of value • Determine the cost of each incremental unit of value provided by the new technology vs. its comparator	• As above	• Examine one medical benefit common to both interventions • Measured in natural units reflecting longevity (e.g., life-years gained) or morbidity (e.g., clinical event prevented) outcomes	• ICER: Incremental cost-effectiveness ratio
Cost-utility analysis (CUA)	• Idem CEA	• As above	• Examine one or more medical consequences not necessarily common to both interventions • Consequences translated into a common measure, the quality-adjusted life-year (QALY)	• ICUR: Incremental cost-utility ratio
Cost-benefit analysis (CBA)	• Determine the net monetary impact of studied interventions by reviewing both related cost and consequences in monetary units	• As above	• Examine one or more consequences not necessarily common to both interventions • Medical consequences (longevity, morbidity) • Non-medical consequences	• Net monetary benefit

NA: not applicable

medical costs, as well as non-medical costs related to a disease (Larg et al., 2011) (Table 8.1). The cost-of-illness studies are considered partial economic evaluations because they only investigate the costs and outcomes of a disease without comparing those across two or more interventions (Drummond et al., 2015). However, they still provide important information to decision makers. For instance, they can highlight disease areas with the greatest patient and economic impact and as a result provide directions to policy makers on where to invest. The cost-of-illness studies also offer an understanding of the downstream impact of a disease, which may provide the necessary input to perform more complex economic evaluations.

Analyses that explore both costs and outcomes related to two or more interventions are considered full economic evaluations (Drummond et al., 2015). The types of analyses described hereunder fall in this category. First, for technologies deemed with a similar effectiveness, a cost-minimization analysis (CMA) should be performed. This analysis simply compares the cost related to each option and identifies the less expensive one, i.e., the option that will deliver the same output at a lower cost (Higgins et al., 2012). When the effectiveness of two technologies differs, a cost-consequence analysis (CCA) can be considered. In this case, both costs and consequences are reviewed across the studied technologies and reported in a disaggregated way (Mauskopf et al., 1998). The cost-consequence analysis does not produce one composite measure summarizing the value differential between two technologies, however, as for the cost-of-illness study, it assembles the necessary data to support the conduct of more definitive value assessments such as the cost-effectiveness analyses (CEAs).

The CEAs are the most common type of economic evaluation used to inform decisions in healthcare. It compares a new intervention with an existing alternative, usually the current standard of care, reviewing incremental costs over incremental health benefits (i.e., effectiveness). When an intervention is more effective and less costly than its alternative, it is deemed "dominant," or cost-saving, and its adoption is justified from a cost-effectiveness standpoint. On the contrary, if that intervention is less effective and more costly, it is dominated by the current standard of care which may prevail. However, new health technologies are often both more effective and more costly than their predecessors, in which case a ratio of cost over benefits needs to be calculated. That is, the incremental cost-effectiveness ratios (ICER). More specifically, that composite measure of value represents the cost for each additional unit of value delivered by the new intervention when compared to its alternative. Depending on the decision maker's willingness to pay for that additional unit of value (ICER threshold), the new intervention may or may not be deemed cost-effective. Of note, there is also a less common scenario where a new technology is less effective and less costly than its comparator. In this case, the ICER will also support a decision, but it reflects the health benefit that a decision maker is willing to forfeit in order to generate the savings offered by the new technology (Higgins et al., 2012; Drummond et al., 2015; Lakdawalla et al., 2018).

The costs included in the CEAs, and other economic evaluations, vary depending on the perspective chosen and the expected end user. The second panel on cost-effectiveness in health and medicine recommends carrying and reporting analyses representing both a healthcare and a societal perspective. The healthcare perspective includes formal healthcare costs borne by third-party payers and the patients (e.g., out-of-pocket costs), and the informal healthcare costs such as patient time, caregiver time, and transportation. The societal perspective will in addition include non-healthcare costs such as productivity and social services. For measuring the effectiveness in CEAs, a wide range of patient outcomes translating longevity and morbidity can be considered depending on the condition under study. Those would lead to results such as incremental cost per life-year gained and incremental cost per clinical event prevented (e.g., cardiovascular event, tumor progression). Since CEAs are often modeled over a multi-year time horizon, it is recommended to discount both future costs and benefits as to reflect their present-day value (Sanders et al., 2016).

A common measure of patient benefit is the quality-adjusted life-year (QALY). The economic evaluations using the QALY as the measure of effectiveness are referred to as cost-utility analyses (CUAs), a subset of CEAs. The QALY adjusts the duration of life with the health state utility, i.e., the quality of life experienced by a patient while under a specific health state. This health state utility varies between 0 (quality of life equivalent to death) and 1 (perfect quality of life). CUAs produce an incremental cost-utility ratio (ICUR) representing the cost to gain one additional QALY when using the newer technology instead of its alternative (Higgins et al., 2012). The use of the QALY, as a standard measure of effectiveness, has the advantage of allowing value comparison across health technologies developed for unrelated disease areas. The results can be compiled and ranked in a league table to contrast the performances of various interventions. Of note, for this exercise to be valid, the studies included must have consistent methodologies (e.g., study timeframe, perspective, discounting of costs and benefits) (Mauskopf, 2003; Wilson, 2019).

The last type of economic analysis presented in this section is the cost-benefit analysis (CBA). As for the other economic evaluations, the CBA examined both the costs and benefits associated with the studied interventions. However, the benefits are converted into monetary units. The output of this analysis is the net monetary benefit and is obtained by subtracting the cost of implementing an intervention (input) from the cost associated with its benefits (output). An intervention is favored in presence of a positive net monetary benefit. Due to the challenges in valuing certain health outcomes (e.g., survival) in monetary terms, CBA are less commonly used. However, because the measure of value (i.e., the net monetary benefit), is expressed in a monetary unit, and not in natural unit (e.g., life year, QALY, health event), it allows the comparison of interventions across healthcare and non-healthcare sectors which may present an advantage for government stakeholders handling cross-sectorial decisions (Higgins et al., 2012; Drummond et al., 2015).

During the last decades, the emergence of HTA authorities and the increasing reliance on economic evaluations to inform healthcare decisions have forced the field of health economics to constantly refine its standards and methodological approaches. We provided above an overview of the categories of economic evaluations and context for their use, but important methodological aspects related to conducting such analyses were not presented. This includes topics such as the choice of comparators, study perspective, analytical approaches (trial-based evaluation vs. economic model), valuing and measuring cost, benefits, and patient preferences (utility), and testing for the robustness of the results (sensitivity analyses). Specialized references (Drummond et al., 2015; Sanders et al., 2016) are available to guide the analysts in the conduct, reporting, and appraisal of the economic analyses.

8.2 Outcome Assessment and Analysis of Outcomes

This section presents and illustrates methods that are commonly used to analyze outcomes variables for health economics outcomes and population health research, e.g., via observational real-world data (RWD) studies, survey sampling studies, non-interventional studies, or pragmatic clinical trials based on RWD (de Vet et al., 2010).
In clinical research

> an outcome assessment… is the measuring instrument that provides a rating or score (categorical or continuous) that is intended to represent some aspect of the patient's health status. Outcome assessments are used to define efficacy endpoints when developing a therapy for a disease or condition. Most efficacy endpoints are based on specified clinical assessments of patients. When clinical assessments are used as clinical trial outcomes, they are called clinical outcome assessments (COAs).
>
> *Walton et al., 2015*

There are four types of COA.

- Patient-reported outcomes (PROs)
- Clinician-reported outcomes (ClinROs)
- Observer-reported outcomes (ObsROs)
- Performance outcomes (PerfOs)

For continuous random variables, descriptive statistics (e.g., minimum, first quartile, median, third quartile, and maximum), as well as graphical displays such as histogram and boxplot, can be used. Hypothesis tests (e.g., two-sample t-test and the one-way or two-way analysis of variance, or their non-parametric counterparts like the Wilcoxon rank-sum test, Kruskal-Wallis test and Friedman tests) are frequently applied.

Among continuous variables and in particular, the cost variable tends to be skewed and bimodal in a mixture of zeros and is positively skewed towards its tail. There are ways to model cost variables using generalized linear models (GLMs) with various link functions and the two-part model. Alternatively, GLMs have been frequently used (Buntin and Zaslavsky, 2004). It was found that the following four modes performed similarly well, including (1) the ordinary least squares model with two smearing factors to correct for heteroscedasticity; (2) constant variance one-part generalized linear model (GLM); (3) two-part generalized linear models; (4) variance proportional to mean (e.g., Poisson-like) GLM model. Furthermore, transformation of the independent and outcome variables may be considered (Mullahy, 1998).

For discrete random variables, on the other hand, descriptive statistics (e.g., count and proportion), as well as graphical displays (e.g., bar diagram and pie chart), can be used. Hypothesis tests (e.g., two-sample t-test and the analysis of variance) are also frequently used. For example, ordinal Likert scale based on discrete data is often used in survey instruments. To draw inferences, either the mean or median is used. However, it is difficult to interpret a factional number as a mean value between two integer ratings, while the median can be too crude for visual comparisons.

Responder analysis of patient reported outcomes that can arise from survey questionnaires is about within-group change over time, while clinically important difference (CID) is about between-group change (Norman et al., 2003; Cappelleri et al., 2013). Both changes are useful for interpreting and analyzing a patient-reported outcome (PRO). The Food and Drug Administration (FDA, 2009) recommends plotting cumulative distribution functions (c.d.f.) to help interpret the clinical relevance of a PRO. For example, the cumulative distribution on change scores can be plotted by treatment and compared between treatment groups. We highlight distribution- and anchor-based methods for the CID and evaluate the influence of correlation between the target PRO and its anchor, which is an external measure with a clear interpretation and appreciably correlated with the PRO measure, on the resulting CID estimates from an empirical data set and a simulated one. Typically, the investigators may be interested in exploring what factors (correlation, standard deviation, methodology) influence estimates of what is an important difference between groups. In this review article, we examine the types of methods, distributed and anchor based, for estimating a CID.

A distribution-based method may first be examined and estimates a CID as a score corresponding to a priori benchmark values for standardized deviation units, defined as the difference in mean changes divided by a measure of variability (Cohen, 1988; Cappelleri et al., 2013). For a two-treatment group comparison, there are three common distribution-based approaches: (1) effect size (ES) with the difference in treatment group means divided by the pooled standard deviation (SD) of the baseline scores; (2) ES with the difference in treatment group means divided by the pooled SD of follow-up scores; and (3) standardized response mean with the difference between the two mean changes from baseline divided by the pooled SD of the change from baseline. Distribution-based method estimates a meaningful importance difference as a surrogate or proxy to CID by using ES in terms of SD units.

The most widely cited benchmark values for Cohen's (1988) ES are 0.2, 0.5, and 0.8, indicating small, medium, and large ES, respectively. Since we are looking for a meaningful important difference where the CID may represent a minimum important difference (MID), we can consider ES between 0.2 and 0.5, or more extreme. Then, CID=0.5×SD, which provides an estimate of the CID to be one half of the measure of variability measured by the SD (SE). The CID may generally be defined as a score between a small and moderate effect size. Effect sizes are calculated as follows: 0.2×SD, 0.5×SD, or 0.8×SD at baseline (ES) and the change from baseline (standardized response mean). Researchers may wish to use half of the standard deviation. Here and with the distribution-based approach in general, the focus is on meaningful difference, not CID. Distribution-based approach is strictly a statistical approach, so CID cannot be performed prospectively.

The best way to proceed in practice is to take an anchor-based approach, take its estimated CID along with a measure of variability (e.g., SD of baseline score), and then calculate retrospectively what the effect size is, i.e., CID divided by the SD of baseline scores in Y.

The CID generally referred to as the meaningful important difference that serves, and it is more general than the concept of the minimum important difference (MID) often found in the PRO literature (Salaffi et al., 2004; Rejas et al., 2008; King, 2011). Thus, in this framework, the distribution-based approach covers a meaningful difference but not a clinically important one. Such a meaningful difference is taken subsequently as an estimate of a CID. One may interpret this method as defining CID as being a value that is distinguishable from background noise or variability.

An anchor-based method is presented and defines responders using an anchor measure correlated with the PRO measure of interest. An anchor can have several response categories such as major deterioration, some deterioration, little deterioration, no change, little improvement, some improvement, and major improvement. The anchor-based method involves mean changes on the PRO with respect to response categories of an anchor, which includes a mean-based method and a receiver operating characteristic curve (ROC)

TABLE 8.2

Sensitivity and Specificity Values

Outcome Variable	Minimum Responder	No Change
Improved	True Positive (TP)	False Positive (FP)
No change or Worsened	False Negative (FN)	True Negative (TN)

Sensitivity = True Positive Fraction=TP / (TP + FN).
Specificity = True Negative Fraction=TN / (TN + FP).
CID is computed at the maximal Youden's Index, YI=Sensitivity+ Specificity-1.

method, (Table 8.2), across various thresholds, to optimally differentiate between responders and non-responders (Zou et al., 2011; Farrar et al., 2006).

An anchor is an external predictor that, ideally, is easy to interpret and bears an appreciable correlation with the target measure of interest. There are different types of anchors. For example, one type is retrospective and can be based on a cross-sectional assessment asked at the end of the study; another type is serial and can be based on a longitudinal assessment of the change in the same measure taken at two time points at baseline and follow-up, respectively.

Definitions and algorithms for evaluating medication adherence and persistence, as well as time to discontinuity of medication uses, and switch to another medication may be conducted. See, for example, the International Society for Pharmacoeconomics and Outcomes Research's (ISPOR, 2022) Medication Adherence and Persistence Special Interest Group with several articles. Finally, for multivariable analysis, it is important and recommended to pre-specify the covariates of interest in the protocol and analysis plan (Agency for Healthcare Research and Quality, 2020). With two or more parallel groups of medications or non-medication interventions, including a placebo arm, it is often needed to match patients systematically, such as using propensity score matching.

In several prior monographs, descriptive and multivariate statistical methods for health economics and outcome research based on RWD and aggregate data analyses are described in detail (Zou et al., 2011, Cappelleri et al., 2013 and Alemayehu et al., 2018).

Remarks

The use of economic evaluations and PROs are key levers to achieving value-based healthcare (Tsevat et al., 2018). However, on this journey to balance patient access to promising technologies with the need for system efficiency, additional factors must be considered in decision making beyond the quantitative assessment of clinical and economic value. An area of growing importance is the patient involvement in the health technology assessment (HTA) process (Groenewoud et al., 2019; Mühlbacher, 2015). This allows patient experience to be captured in order to validate the outcomes that matter to specific patient groups or sub-groups and to identify educational or other patient needs.

There is evidence demonstrating a positive impact of such engagement to improve the robustness and acceptability of policy recommendations (Single et al., 2019). Despite such benefits, this is still an emerging practice and further guidance is necessary to ensure a consistent approach to engaging patients and generating evidence (Wale et al., 2017; Hunter et al., 2018).

Looking ahead, there are opportunities for authorities to strengthen their partnerships with patients to deliver an efficient patient-centered healthcare.

Disclaimer

Jean-Pascal Roussy is a former employee of Upjohn, a Division of Pfizer, and Viatris. Kelly H. Zou is an employee of Viatris, merged between Upjohn, a Division of Pfizer, and Mylan. The views expressed are the authors' own and do not necessarily represent those of their employer or employers. The authors appreciate the editorial support from Arghya Bhattacharya and Aswin Kumar A of Viatris.

References

Agency for Healthcare Research and Quality. Developing a protocol for Observational Comparative Effectiveness Research: A User's Guide. 2013. https://effectivehealthcare.ahrq.gov/products/observational-cer-protocol/research, Accessed 29 October 2020.

Alemayehu D, Cappelleri JC, Emir B, Zou KH. Statistical Topics in Health Economics and Outcomes Research. Chapman and Hall/CRC Press: Boca Raton, FL, USA, 2018.

Buntin MB, Zaslavsky AM. Too much ado about two-part models and transformation? Comparing methods of modeling Medicare expenditures. J Health Econ. 2004 May; 23(3): 525–542.

Cappelleri JC, Zou KH, Bushmakin AG, Alvir JMaJ, Alemayahu D, Symonds T. Patient-Reported Outcomes: Measurement, Implementation and Interpretation. Chapman & Hall/CRC Press: Boca Raton, FL, USA, 2013.

Cohen J. Statistical power analysis for the behavioural sciences (2nd Ed). Lawrence Erlbaum Associates, New York, 1988.

de Vet HCW, Terwee, CB, Mokkink LB, Knol DL. Measurement in Medicine. Cambridge University Press, New York, 2010.

Drummond MF, Sculpher MJ, Claxton K et al. 2015. Chapter 2. Making decisions in health care. In *Methods for the economic evaluation of health care programmes*, Fourth editions, p. 19–40. Oxford University Press

Drummond MF, Sculpher MJ, Claxton K et al. 2015. Chapter 3. Critical assessment of economic evaluation. In *Methods for the economic evaluation of health care programmes*, Fourth editions, p. 41–76. Oxford University Press

Farrar JT, Dworkin RH, Max MB. Use of the cumulative proportion of responders analysis graph to present pain data over a range of cut-off points: making clinical trial data more understandable. J Pain Symptom Manage. 2006; 31: 369–377.

Food and Drug Administration. U.S. Department of Health and Human Services,. Guidance for industry. Patient-reported outcome measures: use in medical product development to support labeling claims. 2009. www.fda.gov/regulatory-information/search-fda-guidance-documents/patient-reported-outcome-measures-use-medical-product-development-support-labeling-claims (Accessed 29 October 2022).

Groenewoud AS, Westert GP, Kremer JAM. Value based competition in health care's ethical drawbacks and the need for a values-driven approach. BMC Health Services Research. 2019; 19: 256.

Higgins AM, Harris AH. Health economic methods: cost-minimization, cost-effectiveness, cost-utility, and cost-benefit evaluations. Crit Care Clin. 2012 Jan; 28(1): 11–24.

Hunter A, Facey K, Thomas V et al. EUPATI Guidance for Patient Involvement in Medicines Research and Development: Health Technology Assessment. Front. Med. 2018; 5: 231.

International Society for Pharmacoeconomics and Outcomes Research (ISPOR). Medication Adherence and Persistence Special Interest Group. 2022. www.ispor.org/member-groups/special-interest-groups/medication-adherence-and-persistence. (Accessed 29 October 2022).

Kernick DP. Introduction to health economics for the medical practitioner. Postgrad Med J. 2003 Mar; 79(929): 147–50. doi: 10.1136/pmj.79.929.147. PMID: 12697913; PMCID: PMC1742631.

King MT. A point of minimal important difference (MID): a critique of terminology and methods. Expert Rev Pharmacoecon Outcomes Res. 2011; 11: 171–184.

Lakdawalla DN, Doshi JA, Garrison LP et al. Defining Elements of Value in Health Care – A Health Economics Approach: An ISPOR Special Task Force Report. Value Health. 2018; 21: 131–139.

Larg A, Moss JR. Cost-of-illness studies: a guide to critical evaluation. PharmacoEconomics. 2011 Aug; 29(8): 653–671.

Mauskopf J, Rutten F, Schonfeld W. Cost-effectiveness league tables: valuable guidance for decision makers? PharmacoEconomics. 2003; 21(14): 991–1000.

Mauskopf JA, Paul JE, Grant DM et al. The role of cost-consequence analysis in healthcare decision-making. Pharmacoeconomics. 1998 Mar; 13(3): 277–288.

Mühlbacher AC. Patient-centric HTA: different strokes for different Folks. Expert Rev Pharmacoeconomics Outcomes Res. 2015; 15(4): 591–597.

Mullahy J. Much ado about two: reconsidering retransformation and the two-part model in health econometrics. J Health Econ. 1998 Jun; 17(3): 247–281.

Norman GR, Sloan JA, Wyrwich KW. Interpretation of changes in health-related quality of life: the remarkable universality of half a standard deviation. Med Care. 2003; 41: 582–592.

Rejas J, Pardo A, Ruiz MA. Standard error of measurement as a valid alternative to minimally important difference for evaluating the magnitude of changes in patient-reported outcomes measures. J Clin Epidemiol. 2008 Apr; 61: 350–356.

Salaffi F, Stancati A, Silvestri CA, Ciapetti A, Grassi W. Minimal clinically important changes in chronic musculoskeletal pain intensity measured on a numerical rating scale. Eur J Pain. 2004; 8: 283–291.

Sanders GD, Neumann PJ, Basu A, et al. Recommendations for Conduct, Methodological Practices, and Reporting of Cost-effectiveness Analyses, Second Panel on Cost-Effectiveness in Health and Medicine. JAMA. 2016; 316(10): 1093–1103.

Single ANV, Facey KM, Livingstone H et al. Stories of Patient Involvement Impact in Health Technology Assessments: A Discussion Paper. Int J Technol Assess Health Care. 2019; 35(4): 266–272.

Tsevat J, Moriates C. Value-Based Health Care Meets Cost-Effectiveness Analysis. Ann Intern Med. 2018; 169: 329–332.

Wale JL, Scott AM, Bertelsen N et al. Strengthening international patient advocacy perspectives on patient involvement in HTA within the HTAi Patient and Citizen Involvement Interest Group – Commentary. Res Involvement Engagement. 2017; 3: 3.

Walton MK, Powers JH 3rd, Hobart J et al. Clinical Outcome Assessments: Conceptual Foundation-Report of the ISPOR Clinical Outcomes Assessment – Emerging Good Practices for Outcomes Research Task Force. Value Health. 2015; 18(6): 741–752. doi:10.1016/j.jval.2015.08.006

Wilson N, Davies A, Brewer N et al. Can cost-effectiveness results be combined into a coherent league table? Case study from one high-income country. Popul Health Metr. 2019 Aug 5; 17(1): 10.

Zou KH, Liu A, Bandos AI, Ohno-Machado L, Rockette HE. Statistical Evaluation of Diagnostic Performance: Topics in ROC Analysis. Chapman and Hall/CRC Press: Boca Raton, FL, USA, 2011.

9

Partnerships and Collaborations

Salman Rizvi and Urooj A. Siddiqui
Viatris

CONTENTS

9.1 The Evolving Healthcare Landscape

The healthcare landscape is constantly changing, thus, compelling pharmaceutical companies to revise their research and development models. Innovation remains at the forefront of the industry's goals; however, the pharmaceutical industry faces numerous challenges that are causing a decline in productivity. Some of these challenges include the high cost and high failure rate of the drug development process; decreasing product pipelines and proprietary assets due to patent expiry and drug withdrawals due to safety concerns; and rising healthcare costs (Khanna, 2012).

In order to stay successful in a consistently evolving market, pharmaceutical companies are embracing partnerships and collaborations as a way of overcoming these challenges (Martinez-Grau & Alvim-Gaston, 2019). Innovative collaboration models, such as public–private partnerships, open innovation models, and industry–academic partnerships, have been crucial for accelerating the healthcare agenda within the industry (Khanna, 2012).

DOI: 10.1201/9781003017523-9

9.2 Partnerships in Healthcare

In the last three decades, pharmaceutical companies have started to move away from the traditional fully integrated business model to an open innovation organizational model that incorporates strategic alliances and partnerships, outsourcing of scientific services and in-licensing. The new model was optimal to develop novel treatments and translate them from bench to bedside. Open innovation was further encouraged by the entry of biotechnology companies into the industry in the 1980s, which acted as intermediates between academic institutions and pharmaceutical companies (Cockburn, 2004; de Vrueh & Crommelin, 2017).

Public-private partnerships are a type of open innovation model that are optimal to transform basic science into clinical value (de Vrueh & Crommelin, 2017; Martinez-Grau & Alvim-Gaston, 2019). This model exploits the expertise of multiple stakeholders, including academia, small and large biopharmaceutical companies, government bodies, regulatory agencies, health foundations and patient organizations. Each private and public stakeholder has a diverse and non-overlapping role in the biomedical research and developmental process (de Vrueh & Crommelin, 2017).

Collaborations between pharmaceutical companies and universities have been around for the last three to four decades and may involve a single academic institution or multi-partner consortia. Policy changes such as the Bayh Dole Act of 1980 enabled licensing of government-sponsored research, thus encouraging these partnerships (de Vrueh & Crommelin, 2017; Yildirim et al., 2016). Universities are driven by the opportunity to contribute and learn about industry research activities, and to gain access to financial and material resources. On the other hand, pharmaceutical companies benefit by gaining access to basic research, and novel ideas, tools and technologies. This partnership additionally helps build brand reputation in the market, and enables utilization of public funding opportunities (de Vrueh & Crommelin, 2017).

Partnerships between pharmaceutical and medical device companies are considered to be one of the top five drivers of growth in these industries (PACK EXPO Healthcare Hub, 2017). Medical device companies provide novel solutions to pharma companies in the aspect of delivery systems for drugs and biologics, and technology for precision medicine (Kubala, 2018). In 2018, GE Healthcare partnered with Roche to set up a precision medicine oncology platform to provide clinical solutions to cancer patients based on advanced analytics (Monegain, 2018). Takeda Pharmaceuticals and Portal Instruments collaborated in 2017 to develop a needle-free delivery system for Takeda's biologics using technology which was developed at the Massachusetts Institute of Technology (MIT) (2017). Therefore, the pharmaceutical industry can expand even further by engaging multiple partners and stakeholders to treat diseases in a timely and effective manner (Kubala, 2018).

Some of the biggest partnerships are those between multiple private companies and represent a private-private partnership. In the field of research and development, joining forces aims to reduce costs and utilizes the expertise of each partner (Allport, 2013). Merck Sharp & Dohme (MSD) have partnered with Taiho Pharmaceutical and Astex Pharmaceuticals to investigate small molecule inhibitors against various drug targets including the KRAS oncogene (Smith, 2020).

As the healthcare industry grows and develops, pharmaceutical companies have started focusing on patient centricity. While the traditional view of patient-focused care placed the patient at the centre of service delivery, the current idea is inclusion of the patient in an active decision-making role. This has fueled partnerships between pharmaceutical companies and patient associations, thus empowering patients to have a more collaborative relationship with hospitals, healthcare providers and policy makers. These partnerships are driven by the needs and experiences of the patient and understanding the patient journey during the course of a disease (du Plessis et al., 2017).

9.3 Collaboration Amidst the COVID-19 Crisis

The emerging COVID-19 pandemic not only threatens the global healthcare landscape, but also the progress made in tackling communicable and non-communicable diseases (NCDs). The pandemic crisis has called for collaboration between various government agencies, pharmaceutical companies, funding agencies, healthcare professionals, social workers, etc., to communicate with the public and halt the further spread of the SARS-CoV-2 virus. Further, partnerships are essential for the development of therapeutic molecules and vaccines against this virus (Chakraborty et al., 2020).

Interest in fair and equitable access to a potential COVID-19 vaccine has stimulated collaboration between global agencies and more than 150 countries. The COVAX facility is a key part of the global collaboration initiated for the development and access of COVID-19 tests, treatments and vaccines. COVAX is jointly led by Gavi, the international public-private partnership, the foundation Coalition for Epidemic Preparedness Innovations (CEPI) and the World Health Organization (WHO). As a part of the COVAX mechanism, 75 countries have agreed to finance vaccine distribution in their own country, as well as support up to 90 low-income countries through donations. This represents more than 60% of the global population. This partnership ensures that poorer nations are also provided with access to treatments and vaccines, unlike the situation seen during the H1N1 pandemic 10 years ago (WHO, 2020b).

Another public-private partnership, Accelerating COVID-19 Therapeutic Interventions and Vaccines (ACTIV), brings together the United States (US) National Institutes of Health (NIH) with other government agencies and departments, academia representatives, philanthropic organizations, biopharmaceutical companies and the foundation for the NIH. This partnership engages the expertise of stakeholders from multiple sectors. Though its focus is on vaccine trials in the US, its COVID-19 Prevention Networks involve coordination with the WHO, CEPI and other global partners, and have a global agenda (Corey et al., 2020).

The COVID-19 pandemic has slowed down the fight against NCDs. Screening and rehabilitation services for the treatment of hypertension, diabetes, cancer and cardiovascular complications have been disrupted, mainly due to the diversion of resources towards COVID-19 (WHO, 2020a). However, the pandemic situation has also seen partnership models emerge to converge expertise from the public and private sector in order to manage NCDs, such as Project chAnGE (Alessandro Monaco & Shaantanu Donde, 2020; Palmer et al., 2020). This partnership, spearheaded by the European Commission, aims to address the challenges of healthy ageing in NCD patients in Europe. This partnership focuses on adherence, integrated care and preventing functional decline in elderly patients with NCDs (Alessandro Monaco & Shaantanu Donde, 2020).

9.4 Innovation in a Post-Pandemic World

In a post-pandemic or an endemic world, the coordination between the public and private sector is pivotal to tackling NCDs. Learnings from the COVID-19 situation have presented opportunities to manage NCDs by leveraging digital health technologies and telemedicine. These solutions will enable access to healthcare resources and services, educational information as well as virtual monitoring from healthcare professionals. The implementation of this model will require a concerted effort from the public and private sector, including organizing awareness and education campaigns, providing access to digital tools to communicate with healthcare professionals, improving healthcare communication to the public and access to local support activities (Palmer et al., 2020).

With the advent and expansion of digital technologies in a post-COVID-19 world, digital partnerships will be a necessity for growth. Advances in digital technology have prompted technology companies, such as Apple, Google and Amazon, just to name a few, besides healthcare technology, insurance, big data and artificial intelligence companies, to experiment with entering the healthcare industry (Champagne et al., 2015). In 2018, e-commerce giant, Amazon teamed up with JPMorgan Chase and Berkshire Hathaway to reduce healthcare costs for employees in the US, but the joint vendure Heaven was not able to fulfil its purpose to disrupt the healthcare industry (Landi, 2021) Amazon Care, the healthcare program for its employees, was launched in 2019 (Farr, 2019; LaVito & Cox, 2018). A partnership between Amazon and the United Kingdom's National Health Service (NHS) aims to provide health information to people through Amazon's smart speaker, Alexa (Downey, 2019). Amazon has also acquired the online pharmacy startup PillPack in an effort to enter into the pharmaceutical distribution market (2018a). In an attempt to compete with Amazon, the shipping and supply chain management company, United Parcel Service (UPS) in partnership with Merck, aims to expand their distribution agreement to a health service that brings clinicians to deliver vaccines to patients in their homes (Truong, 2019).

In order to stay competitive, pharmaceutical companies have begun collaborating with companies providing digital solutions and innovations. Some of the opportunities for collaboration include personalized healthcare with the advent of digital sensors and services tailored to the needs of the patient, digital communication channels between healthcare providers and patients, data-driven advanced analytics and automated processes, among others (Champagne et al., 2015). For example, partnered with the digital diagnostics company Ellume Limited to develop digital products targeting respiratory health Biospace, 2018). Roche is collaborating with Qualcomm Life, a subsidiary of the wireless technology company Qualcomm, to improve remote monitoring and engagement between healthcare professionals and chronic disease patients (Qualcomm, 2015).

In the last decade, the wearable technology market has rapidly grown and expanded to include wristbands, glasses, in-ear monitors and electronic shirts (Cheung et al., 2018). However, patients utilizing these technologies may lack the education and understanding of their functioning and the implication of the data output (Knowles et al., 2018). The Bristol-Myers Squibb (2019) and Pfizer Alliance has partnered with Fitbit to develop educational content and guidance for patients at risk for atrial fibrillation. This partnership rests on the Food and Drug Administration's (FDA)clearance of atrial fibrillation detection software on Fitbit devices (2019b).

Partnerships in the pharmaceutical industry provide opportunities for drug development and innovation to advance at rates much higher than pharma companies could accomplish independently. These collaborations provide efficiency and cost-saving in the development of innovative medicine, thus improving clinical outcomes by utilizing a patient-centric approach (Yildirim et al., 2016).

Summary

Pharmaceutical companies have started moving away from the traditional fully integrated business model to an open innovation organizational model. Despite challenges, the path forward is to adopt an innovative collaborative approach such as public–private partnerships, and industry–academic partnerships. The COVID-19 pandemic has compromised the fight against NCDs due to the diversion of resources towards COVID-19. Though care of NCD is of paramount importance partnerships for the development of vaccines against this virus have taken a centre stage globally. With the advent of digital technology in a post-COVID-19 world, digital partnerships will be a necessity for growth and to maximize patient access.

Disclaimer

Salman Rizvi and Urooj A. Siddiqui Viatris are employees of Viatris, merged between Upjohn, a Division of Pfizer, and Mylan. The views expressed are the authors' own and do not necessarily represent those of their employer or employers. The authors appreciate the editorial support from Arghya Bhattacharya and Aswin Kumar A of Viatris.

References

Alessandro, M., Shaantanu, D. 2020. Time to accelerate progress on healthy ageing. *Politico.*

Allport, S. 2013. All Change for Pharma and Biotech Partnerships. *Phenestra White Paper.*

Biospace. Strategic partnership announced with global healthcare company GSK. 2018. www.biospace.com/article/strategic-partnership-announced-with-global-healthcare-company-gsk (Accessed on March 30, 2022).

BiotechDispatch. Anteo updates on partnership with Ellume. 2019. https://biotechdispatch.com.au/news/anteo-updates-on-partnership-with-ellume (Accessed on March 30, 2022).

Bristol Myers Squibb. The Bristol-Myers Squibb-Pfizer Alliance and Fitbit Collaborate to Address Gaps in Atrial Fibrillation Detection with the Aim of Accelerating Diagnosis. 2019. https://news.bms.com/news/partnering/2019/The-Bristol-Myers-Squibb-Pfizer-Alliance-and-Fitbit-Collaborate-to-Address-Gaps-in-Atrial-Fibrillation-Detection-with-the-Aim-of-Accelerating-Diagnosis/default.aspx (Accessed on March 30, 2022).

Business Wire. Amazon to Acquire PillPack. 2018. www.businesswire.com/news/home/20180628005614/en/Amazon-to-Acquire-PillPack (Accessed on March 30, 2022).

Chakraborty, C., Sharma, A.R., Sharma, G., Bhattacharya, M., Saha, R.P., Lee, S.-S. 2020. Extensive Partnership, Collaboration, and Teamwork is Required to Stop the COVID-19 Outbreak. *Archives of Medical Research.*

Champagne, D., Hung, A., Leclerc, O. 2015. The road to digital success in pharma. *McKinsey White Paper.*

Cheung, C.C., Krahn, A.D., Andrade, J.G. 2018. The Emerging Role of Wearable Technologies in Detection of Arrhythmia. *Can J Cardiol*, 34(8), 1083–1087.

Cockburn, I.M. 2004. The changing structure of the pharmaceutical industry. *Health Affairs*, 23(1), 10–22.

Corey, L., Mascola, J.R., Fauci, A.S., Collins, F.S. 2020. A strategic approach to COVID-19 vaccine R&D. *Science*, 368, 948–950.

de Vrueh, R.L.A., Crommelin, D.J.A. 2017. Reflections on the Future of Pharmaceutical Public-Private Partnerships: From Input to Impact. *Pharmaceutical Research*, 34(10), 1985–1999.

Downey, A. 2019. Alexa will see you now: NHS partners with Amazon, Vol. 2020, Digitalhealth.

du Plessis, D., Sake, J.-K., Halling, K., Morgan, J., Georgieva, A., Bertelsen, N. 2017. Patient centricity and pharmaceutical companies: is it feasible? *Therapeutic Innovation & Regulatory Science*, 51(4), 460–467.

Farr, C. 2019. Amazon launches Amazon Care, a virtual medical clinic for employees, Vol. 2020, CNBC.

Khanna, I. 2012. Drug discovery in pharmaceutical industry: productivity challenges and trends. *Drug Discovery Today*, 17(19), 1088–1102.

Knowles, B.H., Smith, A., Poursabzi-Sangdeh, F., Lu, D., Alabi, H. 2018. Attending to the Problem of Uncertainty in Current and Future Health Wearables. *Communications of the ACM*. pp. 1–6.

Kubala, M. 2018. How pharma and medtech collaborations fuel progress, Vol. 2020, Prescouter.

Landi H. There were plenty of red flags that spelled the demise of Amazon, JPMorgan healthcare venture, experts say. Fierce Healthcare. 2021. www.fiercehealthcare.com/tech/these-are-red-flags-spelled-haven-s-demise-according-to-industry-experts (Accessed on March 30, 2022).

LaVito, A., Cox, J. 2018. Amazon, Berkshire Hathaway, and JPMorgan Chase to partner on US employee health care, Vol. 2020, CNBC.

Martinez-Grau, M.A., Alvim-Gaston, M. 2019. Powered by Open Innovation: Opportunities and Challenges in the Pharma Sector. *Pharmaceutical Medicine*, 33(3), 193–198.

Massachusetts Insitute of Technology. Startup's needle-free drug injector gets commercialization deal. 2017. https://news.mit.edu/2017/startup-needle-free-drug-injector-gets-commercialization-deal-1208. (Accessed on March 30, 2022).

Monegain, B. 2018. GE Healthcare partners with Roche to build precision medicine oncology platform, Vol. 2020, Healthcare IT News.

PACK EXPO Healthcare Hub. 2017. 5 reasons for growth in the pharmaceutical and medical device industries, Vol. 2020.

Palmer, K., Monaco, A., Kivipelto, M., Onder, G., Maggi, S., Michel, J.-P., Prieto, R., Sykara, G., Donde, S. 2020. The potential long-term impact of the COVID-19

outbreak on patients with non-communicable diseases in Europe: consequences for healthy ageing. *Aging Clinical and Experimental Research*, 32(7), 1189–1194.
Qualcomm. Roche and Qualcomm Collaborate to Innovate Remote Patient Monitoring. 2015. www.qualcomm.com/news/releases/2015/01/29/roche-and-qualcomm-collaborate-innovate-remote-patient-monitoring (Accessed on March 30, 2022).
Smith, A. 2020. MSD enlists Otsuka units Taiho and Astex to develop KRAS therapies, Vol. 2020, PharmaTimes online.
Truong, K. 2019. Report: UPS to launch healthcare delivery service as competition with Amazon heats up, Vol. 2020, MedCity News.
United Nations. COVID-19 threatens to undo global health progress. 2020. https://news.un.org/en/story/2020/05/1064022 (Accessed on March 30, 2022).
World Health Organization. 2020a. COVID-19 significantly impacts health services for noncommunicable diseases, World Health Organization. Geneva.
World Health Organization. 2020b. More than 150 countries engaged in COVID-19 vaccine global access facility, World Health Organization. Geneva/London.
Yildirim, O., Gottwald, M., Schüler, P., Michel, M.C. 2016. Opportunities and Challenges for Drug Development: Public-Private Partnerships, Adaptive Designs and Big Data. *Frontiers in Pharmacology*, **7**, 461–461.

10

Global Perspective: China Big Data Collaboration to Improve Patient Care

[1] Zhi Xia Xie, [1] Jim Z. Li, [2] Yvonne Huang, [1] Olive Jin, [1] Wei Yu, and [1] Kelly H. Zou

[1] *Viatris,* [2]*Sanofi China*

CONTENTS

10.1 Big Data and Real-World Evidence in China

For medical researchers serving in industry, government, and academia around the world, real-world data (RWD), big data, and digital capabilities and technologies must be enabled and elevated globally, especially when randomized controlled trials (RCTs) become increasingly costly. There are tremendous opportunities around the world to gain medical insights through Real-World Evidence (RWE) and big data outside RCTs. There is a large population who can benefit from medical breakthroughs that can change patients' lives in developing countries in Asia including China, as well as Latin America, Africa and the Middle East. For example, the prevalence of Hypertension (high blood pressure) in China is quite variable by examining the literature (Clarivate, 2021), ranging from 19.8% for adults to 60.6% for those aged 40 or above (Table 10.1).

The expansion of the middle class, the desire for quality medicines and services, and the rise in the morbidity and mortality of non-communicable diseases (NCDs), commonly known as chronic diseases, are the realities that these regions must face every day (Zou et al., 2019; Zou et al., 2020a). Their

DOI: 10.1201/9781003017523-10

TABLE 10.1

Prevalence Rates of Hypertension in China Based on Literature Review via Incidence and Prevalence Database

Age Group (years)	Prevalence Rate (%)	Prevalence Number	Population*
18+	23.2	255,494,251	1,101,268,324
18+	19.8	218,051,128	1,101,268,324
35+	37.2	278,375,632	748,321,592
35 to 75	36.9	258,385,052	700,230,494
35 to 75	44.7	313,003,031	700,230,494
40+	57.3	372,661,647	650,369,367
40+	60.6	394,123,836	650,369,367

increasing needs for quality medicines and services necessitate researchers to conduct more research and generate more evidence, leading to solutions in their populations to help them access optimal and effective medicines and services (The Economist, Intelligence Unit., 2018). Furthermore, the advances in information technologies (IT) and telecommunication infrastructures also drastically enable a massive amount of RWD generated from many sources outside the RCT framework.

Besides medical research, RWD also increasingly plays an important role in patient care. For example, tele-medicines and internet hospitals are on the rise and becoming an increasingly important part of the healthcare system, as is timely development of new medicines and medical services via cutting-edge innovation, especially during the COVID-19 pandemic and afterwards (Hassan et al., 2020). Furthermore, more and more hospitals participate in eHealth networks. Digital innovation can be an efficient way to improve the capability of physicians, helping to guide patients with NCDs to receive individualized treatments and disease management. Data are also useful for evidence generation to monitor healthcare quality and to evaluate the effectiveness of various interventions. Thus, countries with rapid economic growth and well-developed IT infrastructures are ripe with opportunities, and China has put big data for medical research onto roadmaps as a high priority (Zou et al., 2020a).

Developing the resource for and emphasizing the use of RWD in health and medicine is a national priority in China. A recent article written about big data reads as follows:

> In June 2016, the State Council of China issued an official notice on the development and use of big data in the healthcare sector. The council acknowledged that big data in health and medicine were a strategic national resource and their development could improve healthcare in China, and it set out programmatic development goals, key tasks, and an organizational framework.
>
> *Zhang et al., 2018*

Thus, collaborations and partnerships based on big data have been formed in various geographical regions, provinces, cities, and districts.

RWD sources can range from electronic health records (EHR), insurance claims, disease registries, surveys, medical devices, digital apps, and beyond. To fully realize RWD's potential value and allow for better collaboration, data from various sources need to be pooled and linked into big data. However, there are unique challenges there, including data integration and access, interoperability, standardization, quality control, and privacy protection (Figure 10.1). All these necessitate national and international guidance and standards to coordinate and manage. In China, for example, the National Medical Products Administration (NMPA) published a new guidance document "Announcement on the Guidelines for RWE to Support Drug Development and Review" (China National Medical Products Administration, 2020) and RWD Used in Medical Device Clinical Evaluation (Trial Implementation)" (National Medical Products Administration, 2020). Furthermore, the NMPA has issued a guidance on RWE among pediatric patients (Pharma to market, 2020; NMPA, 2020). The US Food and Drug Administration (FDA) has issued RWE guidance documents (U.S. Food and Drug Administration, 2020).

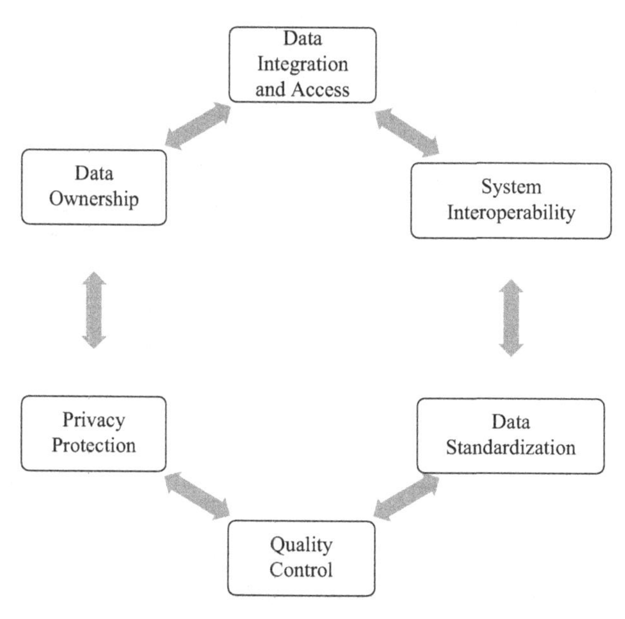

FIGURE 10.1
Challenges of big data and real-world data.

10.2 Digital Innovation During and Post-Pandemic

The healthcare innovation has been advancing much faster in the last two years due to the urgency of the COVID-19 pandemic, where breakthroughs are urgently needed and thereby rapidly adapted via integrated public and private health care systems by a range of healthcare professionals (Heller et al., 2019). Government policies, healthcare accessibility and quality assurance infrastructures must all adapt to the rapidly arriving RWD. Such data, along with data from RCTs, can help develop new therapies and evaluate the outcomes of new interventions.

A major barrier to rapid use RWD for health-care innovation during COVID-19 pademic is access to RWD due to the many diverse data sources and repositories. An additional challenge is to use RWD in support of precision-medicine solutions tailored towards the specific vulnerable patient populations such as the elderly and patients with pre-existing comorbid NCDs, since both advanced age and comorbid conditions drastically increase the severity and mortality of COVID-19.

Data translators, who are like shepherds with subject-matter expert knowledge, as well as data scientists, are needed (Henke N et al., 2018). For example, how to put a complex set of data together, efficiently and accurately, within and across complex healthcare information systems, to improve diagnoses, treatment and follow-up is both challenging and impactful. Chinese characters may make variables and formats in databases harder to standardize, as well as natural language processing. Because of the increased data and privacy protections, institutions tend to have their data with diverse data formats sitting in patient registries without being standardized and connected (Sun X et al., 2018).

Data-driven and data-savvy researchers can and must make a meaningful and impactful contribution to combat fatal diseases during the COVID-19 pandemic. Their skillful data-related capabilities and expertise are critical in generating evidence and gaining insights from big data (Figure 10.2). Furthermore, for digital and technological innovations that can target therapies and optimal treatment strategies, it is imperative to foster multidisciplinary collaborations and partnerships (Zou et al., 2020b).

Summary

Given the advances of data science, big data and RWD are increasingly playing important roles and are harnessed to advance patient health to generate insights, particularly for potential uses in regulatory settings.

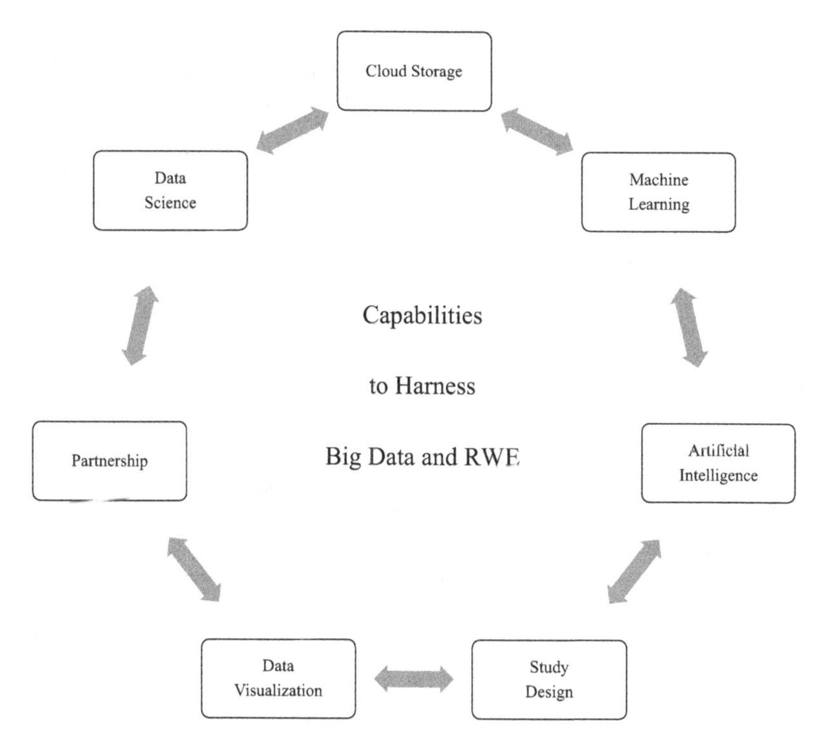

FIGURE 10.2
Capabilities to harness big data and real-world data.

Since NCDs are major diseases to detect and treat in large countries such as China, there are many opportunities with required capabilities. However, barriers in terms of data access and integration still exist, which will need to be dealt with when RWE and digital become important value-added tools for healthcare decision-making.

For future directions, it is imperative to increase the awareness of RWE, build infrastructure for data warehousing and storage, invest in data technologies and data science to harness big data and RWD. Finally, health policy related to data-driven decisions also need to evolve when data become more abundant and in higher quality.

Disclaimer

Zhi Xia Xie, Jim Z. Li, Olive Jin, and Kelly H. Zou are employee of Viatris, merged between Upjohn, a Division of Pfizer, and Mylan. Yvonne Huang is an employee of Sanofi China and a former employee of Upjohn, a Division of Pfizer, and Viatris. Wei Yu a former employee of Upjohn, a Division of Pfizer, and Viatris. The views expressed are the authors' own and do not necessarily represent those of their employers. The chapter was originally published in the International Chinese Statistical Association (ICSA) Bulletin (July issue, 2020) and was reprinted with adaptation via a content-update with permission from the ICSA. The authors also appreciate the editorial support from Arghya Bhattacharya and Aswin Kumar A of Viatris.

References

Clarivate. Hypertension, Incidence & Prevalence Database. 2022. www.tdrdata.com (Accessed July 2021).

Food & Drug Administration. Real World Evidence. 2020. www.fda.gov/science-research/science-and-research-special-topics/real-world-evidence (Accessed November 2, 2021).

Hassan TA, Saenz JE, Ducinskiene D, Imperato J, Zou KH. A confluence of acute and chronic diseases: Risk factors among Covid-19 patients. Significance. 2020. www.significancemagazine.com/science/671-a-confluence-of-acute-and-chronic-diseases-risk-factors-among-covid-19-patients (Accessed November 2, 2020).

Heller DJ, Kumar A, Kishore SP, Horowitz CR, Joshi R, Vedanthan R. Assessment of barriers and facilitators to the delivery of care for noncommunicable diseases by nonphysician health workers in low- and middle-income countries: a systematic review and qualitative analysis. JAMA Netw Open. 2019; 2(12): e1916545.

Henke N, Levine J, McInerney P. You don't have to be a data scientist to fill this must-have analytics role. Harvard Business Review. 2018. https://hbr.org/2018/02/you-dont-have-to-be-a-data-scientist-to-fill-this-must-have-analytics-role (Accessed November 2, 2021).

National Medical Products Administration. NMPA Issued the Announcement on the Guidelines for Real-World Evidence to Support Drug Development and Review (Interim). 2020. http://english.nmpa.gov.cn/2020-01/07/c_456245.htm#:~:text=To%20further%20guide%20and%20standardize,released%20on%20January%207%2C%202020. (Accessed November 2, 2021).

Sun X, Tan J, Tang L, Guo JJ, Li X. Real world evidence: experience and lessons from China. BMJ. 2018; 360: j5262.

The Economist, Intelligence Unit. The cost of silence: cardiovascular disease in Asia: an Economist Intelligence Unit report. The Economist, Intelligence Unit. 2018. https://eiuperspectives.economist.com/healthcare/cost-silence/white-paper/cost-silence-cardiovascular-disease-asia (Accessed November 2, 2021).

Zhang L, Wang H, Li Q, Zhao MH, Zhan QM. Big data and medical research in China. *BMJ* . 2018; 360: j5910. www.bmj.com/content/360/bmj.j5910 (Accessed November 2, 2021).

Zou KH, Li JZ, Hassan TA, Imperato J, Saenz JE, Ducinskiene D. The role of data science and risk assessments during the COVID-19 pandemic. CIO Applications. 2020b.

https://healthcare.cioapplications.com/cxoinsights/the-roles-of-data-science-and-risk-assessments-during-the-covid19-pandemic-nid-5981.html (Accessed November 2, 2021).

Zou KH, Li JZ, Salem LA, Imperato J, Edwards J, Ray A. Harnessing real-world evidence to reduce the burden of noncommunicable disease: health information technology and innovation to generate insights. Health Serv Outcomes Res Methodol. 2020a Nov; 6: 1–13.

Zou KH, Li JZ, Sethi N. Diagnosing and treating noncommunicable diseases around the world. Amstat News. 2019. https://magazine.amstat.org/blog/2019/11/01/diagnosing-and-treating-noncommunicable-diseases-around-the-world (Accessed November 2, 2021).

11

The Future of Patient-Centric Data-Driven Healthcare

Kelly H. Zou,[1] Lobna A. Salem,[1] and Amrit Ray[2]
[1]*Viatris,* [2]*Principled Impact, LLC*

CONTENTS

In *Real-World Evidence in a Patient-Centric Digital Era,* we have discussed the importance of real-world evidence (RWE) in addressing noncommunicable diseases (NCDs) in the areas of medical evidence generation, regulatory approval and access to healthcare (U.S. Food & Drug Administration, 2021). We offer ideas on a future vision for healthcare in which the healthcare community can harness emerging trends in RWE, some of which have accelerated recently in the urgent search for solutions to make an impact on individual patients and public health.

Given the considerable prevalence of NCDs but generally low adherence to treatments and therapies, real-world data (RWD) from outside randomized controlled trials (RCTs) has already proven its added value in advancing global health, particularly from medical evidence, regulatory approval and healthcare access standpoints (Morgan et al., 2020). Given NCDs' destructive effect on patients' and families' lives globally, we must address their burden and impact broadly, urgently and decisively. Early during the coronavirus disease 2019 (COVID) pandemic, Hassan et al. (2020) and Zou et al. (2020b) reviewed NCD-specific comorbidities as COVID-19 risk factors to demonstrate a confluence between NCDs and COVID-19, and Ray (2020) discussed early understandings of the pandemic.

Using evidence generated from multiple RWD sources in multiple global markets, we can map patient journeys to better understand patients' adherence to therapies and measure the outcomes. For example, it is common for

DOI: 10.1201/9781003017523-11

patients with NCDs to have multiple comorbid conditions (Hassan et al., 2020; Zou et al., 2020b). Therefore, harnessing structured and unstructured, as well as quantitative and qualitative, data can help evaluate patients' diagnoses, therapies and prognoses, both holistically and comprehensively. This information can be derived from multiple sources, including digital apps, therapeutics, telehealth records and patient-reported outcomes. As illustrated in Ali et al. (2020) and Rizvi et al. (2020), global partnerships are critical to achieve the successes of multidisciplinary collaborations.

Medical research embraces RWE for multiple uses through patient-centric innovations, electronic survey methods and patient-reported outcomes (PROs). Given that RWE can help understand patients, health conditions, and healthcare resource use (HCRU) beyond RCTs, the use of RWE in a regulatory capacity is gradually increasing. Those of us who generate, interpret, and use evidence must keep in mind the limitations of the source data and analytical approaches. Similar to data obtained from RCTs, transparency of methodology and adoption of best practices are essential. Patients' access to medicines may also be facilitated through the insights from RWE that have enabled patient-diversity in RCTs and RWD, supported pricing and reimbursement decisions by payers, aided business strategies and business development plans from the biopharmaceutical industry, and delivered insights to highlight gaps in market access that have stimulated remedial plans around the world. Government agencies can require or encourage biopharmaceutical companies to obtain adequate medical evidence to develop treatment guidelines, deliver enriched content for medical education and provide critical insights to scientific leaders and subject matter experts. Moreover, RWE has enabled the prioritization of product registration processes, supported regulatory authorities' data queries and provided insights for and value added medicines, such as repurposing medicines and expanding product labels.

Given the above advantages and demonstrated impact from RWE and digital innovations, it is becomingly increasingly important to anticipate and prioritize RWE efforts in the context of registration strategies, data quality and accessibility, and international regulations. For example, early engagement with regulators can support subsequent RWE efforts. Particularly in an era of digital innovation, RWE enables extensive collection, aggregation, analyses, and interpretations to generate useful insights.

Furthermore, regarding the definition and applications of RWE, ensuring the availability of high quality data to feed into artificial intelligence (AI), machine learning (ML) and deep learning (DL) algorithms, as well as steps to ensure ethical research practices, must be carefully considered (Cohen et al., 2017). Value-based care (VBC) can benefit patients, providers, payers, suppliers and society (NEJM Catalyst, 2017). While regulators welcome RWE beyond RCTs, there is still mixed receptiveness and usage across markets on the payer side, e.g., via health technology assessments (Angelis et al.,

2018; Makady et al., 2018). Bottlenecks continue to exist for RWE generation for value-added purposes, e.g., supporting regulatory submissions, new formulations, VBC, and comparative effectiveness research (CER). Therefore, the refinement of analytic algorithms is essential to improve the accuracy and thereby reliability and usability of results.

RWE can be useful in a variety of ways, e.g., patient centricity, patient diversity, medicines regulation, digital innovation via electronic health (eHealth), mobile health (mHealth) and telehealth, and sophisticated algorithms, such as AI, ML and DL. Besides usefulness in harnessing RWE, it can play a role in optimizing RCTs and generating evidence through pragmatic clinical trials (PCTs). Researchers must first ensure that the data obtained are complete and relevant to the condition, patient population, and treatment analyzed. Unstructured data, such as texts, may contain relevant information for only certain sub-populations or information may be entered for some patients but not others. Even structured data pose challenges in the application of RWD analytics and AI since data may have inconsistent terms, different formats between sources, and have incomplete or messy information. These situations can lead to inaccuracies in the analyses and convergence of the algorithms.

Data aggregation poses an equally significant challenge. Legal barriers around data privacy, practical barriers related to data storage, and economic barriers involving the lack of access to care all affect the availability of data to which analytics can be applied. Additional challenges are likely to be encountered in this fast-moving field, especially during the pandemic.

The Data Science discipline has a well-known saying, "garbage in, garbage out." Data standards can cover the quality aspect and the choice of analytic methods. It is also critical to identify multi-disciplinary collaboration that can be skillful in harnessing RWE. If multiple challenges and barriers can be overcome successfully, with data providing sufficient, accurate and comprehensive information, RWE can shorten the timeline for clinical trial design and regulatory approval, as well as uncover patterns in data that would otherwise not be observed.

In summary, RWE and digital methods and tools can be useful in advancing care for NCD patients around the world through end-to-end integration in research and development and medical functions (Zou et al., 2020a; 2020c; 2020d). One example of addressing a public healthcare burden, if applied successfully, can pave the way to broader application in other global health conditions. Throughout this book, we have discussed some key current uses and emerging trends regarding use of RWE to evaluate and enhance NCD care, among other applications. Integrating RWE into NCD care is particularly relevant, given the disproportionate impact of COVID-19 on patients with NCDs. RWE can help better understand the impact of COVID-19 on vulnerable populations, especially elderly patients with NCDs, as well as develop tailored medicine and care plans via precision medicine. The main focus on NCDs is not only due to their serious health burdens, but also the needs to better understand their impact through RWE, given the disproportionate impact of COVID 19 on people living with NCDs. However, the methods presented throughout the book may also be applicable to other communicable diseases beyond NCDs.

Finally, while the use of RWE to capture, combine, standardize, and analyze data is still evolving, it has a potential to support data-driven decision-making to improve global health through patient centricity and patient diversity.

Disclaimer

Kelly H. Zou and Lobna A. Salem are employees of Viatris, merged between Upjohn, a Division of Pfizer, and Mylan. Amrit Ray is an employee of Principled Impact, LLC and a former employee of Upjohn, a Division of Pfizer, and Viatris. The views expressed are the authors' own and do not necessarily represent those of their employer or employers. The authors appreciate the editorial support from Arghya Bhattacharya and Aswin Kumar A of Viatris.

References

Ali R, El Shahawy O, Zou KH, Sherman S, Weitzman M, Ray A. NYU Abu Dhabi and Pfizer Inc.: collaboration drives progress. Amstat News. 2020. https://magazine.amstat.org/blog/2020/04/01/nyu-abu-dhabi-pfizer (Accessed on August 27, 2021).

Angelis A, Lange A, Kanavos P. Using health technology assessment to assess the value of new medicines: results of a systematic review and expert consultation across eight European countries. Eur J Health Econ. 19(1), 123–152 (2018).

Cohen IG, Lynch HF, Vayena E, Gasser U (Eds). Big Data, Health Law, and Bioethics. 2017. Cambridge University Press. 9781107193659_frontmatter.pdf (cambridge.org) (Accessed on August 27, 2021)

Food & Drug Administration. Real-World Evidence. 2021. www.fda.gov/science-research/science-and-research-special-topics/real-world-evidence (Accessed on August 27, 2021).

Hassan TA, Saenz JE, Ducinskiene D, Imperato J, Zou KH. A confluence of acute and chronic diseases: risk factors among Covid-19 patients. Significance. 2020. www.significancemagazine.com/science/671-a-confluence-of-acute-and-chronic-diseases-risk-factors-among-covid-19-patients (Accessed on August 27, 2021).

Makady A, van Veelen A, Jonsson P et al. Using real-world data in health technology assessment (HTA) practice: a comparative study of five HTA agencies. Pharmacoeconomics. 36(3), 359–368 (2018).

Morgan J, Feghali K, Shah S, Miranda W. RWE focus is shifting to R&D, early investments begin to pay off. Deloitte Insights. 2020. www2.deloitte.com/us/en/insights/industry/health-care/real-world-evidence-study.html (Accessed on August 27, 2021).

NEJM Catalyst. What Is Value-Based Healthcare? 2017. https://catalyst.nejm.org/doi/full/10.1056/CAT.17.0558 (Accessed on August 27, 2021).

Ray A. Pharma executive offers thoughts about COVID-19. Amstat News. 2020. https://magazine.amstat.org/blog/2020/08/01/pharma-executive-covid-19 (Accessed on August 27, 2021).

Rizvi S, Majumdar A, Zou KH, Ray A. Partnerships in action: advancing healthcare through collaborative science in emerging markets. CIO Applications. 2020. www.cioapplications.com/cxoinsights/partnerships-in-action-advancing-healthcare-through-collaborative-science-in-emerging-markets-nid-5717.html (Accessed on August 27, 2021).

Zou KH, Imperato J, Ovalle J, Li J, Sethi N, Ray A. Optimizing Patient Care Through AI/ML/DL. PharmaVoice. 2020a. www.pharmavoice.com/wp-content/uploads/PV0620_EnhancedPatientCentricity_WM.pdf?tracker_id=1594684800202 (Accessed on August 27, 2021).

Zou KH, Li JZ, Hassan TA, Imperato J, Saenz JE, Ducinskiene D. The role of data science and risk assessments during the COVID-19 pandemic. CIO Applications. July, 2020b. https://healthcare.cioapplications.com/cxoinsights/the-roles-of-data-science-and-risk-assessments-during-the-covid19-pandemic-nid-5981.html (Accessed on August 27, 2021).

Zou KH, Li JZ, Imperato J, Potkar CN, Sethi N, Edwards J, Ray A. Harnessing Real-World Data for Regulatory Use and Applying Innovative Applications. J Multidiscip Health. 13, 671–679 (2020c).

Zou KH, Li JZ, Salem LA, Imperato J, Edwards J, Ray A. Harnessing real-world evidence to reduce the burden of noncommunicable disease: health information technology and innovation to generate insights. Health Serv Outcomes Res Methodol. 2020d: 1–13.

Index

Note: Page numbers in italics indicate figures and in bold indicate tables on the corresponding pages.

Printed in the United States
by Baker & Taylor Publisher Services